Clóvis Luciano Giacomet (Org)

Knowledge and Practice in Indigenous Health, Education and Culture

Clóvis Luciano Giacomet (Org)

Knowledge and Practice in Indigenous Health, Education and Culture

ScienciaScripts

Imprint
Any brand names and product names mentioned in this book are subject to trademark, brand or patent protection and are trademarks or registered trademarks of their respective holders. The use of brand names, product names, common names, trade names, product descriptions etc. even without a particular marking in this work is in no way to be construed to mean that such names may be regarded as unrestricted in respect of trademark and brand protection legislation and could thus be used by anyone.

Cover image: www.ingimage.com

This book is a translation from the original published under ISBN 978-620-2-04359-5.

Publisher:
Sciencia Scripts
is a trademark of
Dodo Books Indian Ocean Ltd. and OmniScriptum S.R.L publishing group

120 High Road, East Finchley, London, N2 9ED, United Kingdom
Str. Armeneasca 28/1, office 1, Chisinau MD-2012, Republic of Moldova, Europe
Printed at: see last page
ISBN: 978-620-7-22296-4

SUMMARY

AUTHORS 2

PREFACE 5

PRESENTATION 7

1. CHANGES IN THE FOOD HABITS OF INDIGENOUS PEOPLE AND THEIR IMPLICATIONS IN THE HEALTH PROCESS. 8

2. CULTURAL CHANGES RELATED TO HEALTH INSERTED INTO THE INDIGENOUS COMMUNITY THROUGH COEXISTENCE WITH NON-INDIGENOUS SOCIETIES 23

3. NUTRITIONAL STATUS OF INDIGENOUS CHILDREN 37

4. DISEASES ACQUIRED BY THE INDIGENOUS POPULATION THROUGH CONTACT WITH THE NON-INDIGENOUS POPULATION 53

5. INDIGENOUS ORAL HEALTH CARE IN BRAZIL 64

6. THE CONTRIBUTION OF NURSING IN THE CONTROL OF SELF-MEDICATION IN THE INDIGENOUS VILLAGE 80

7. DENTAL CARIES IN INDIGENOUS POPULATIONS IN BRAZIL: AN APPROACH TO IMPROVING ORAL HEALTH 95

8. THE INCLUSION OF INDIGENOUS PEOPLES THROUGH EDUCATION AND WORK: AN APPROACH TO IMPROVING QUALITY OF LIFE 108

9. NURSES AND DIFFERENTIATED CARE FOR INDIGENOUS SOCIETIES 117

10. CULTURAL ORAL HEALTH PREVENTION HABITS OF INDIGENOUS PEOPLES: A HISTORICAL ANALYSIS 147

11. OBESITY IN INDIGENOUS POPULATIONS: AN APPROACH TO IMPROVING QUALITY OF LIFE. 158

12. HEALTH CARE IN THE CARE OF INDIGENOUS WOMEN DURING PREGNANCY 173

13. THE DENTIST'S INTERACTION WITH INDIGENOUS COMMUNITIES AND THE CONSEQUENCES FOR ORAL HEALTH 186

AUTHORS

1. Andrea do Rocio Schneider

Nurse, graduated from Universidade do Centro Oeste - UNICENTRO, 2006. Specialist in occupational nursing at UNINTER in 2010, currently a nurse at the Special Indigenous Secretariat SESAI/MS. E-mail: enfandrea2008@hotmail.com

2. Clóvis Luciano Giacomet

Nurse, graduated from Faculdade de Pato Branco - FADEP. Specialist in the Family Health Program at ESAP. Currently a professor at the Federal University of Amapà - UNIFAP. E-mail: clovisgiacomet@gmail.com

3. Daiza Martins Lopes Goncalves

Dentist. Graduated from Universidade Sao Francisco de Bragança Paulista (USF) 2002, specialist in Endodontics from Universidade Vale do Sapucai (UNIVAS) MG 2015, currently professor of dentistry and Technical Responsible for the dentistry clinic at Faculdade Guairaca in Guarapuava - Paranà and dentist at the Special Indigenous Secretariat, SESAI / MS.

4. Danieli Maria Menon

Nurse. Graduated in Nursing from Guairacà College. Specialist in Urgency and Emergency: from pre-hospital to ICU at Guairacà College. Specialist in Occupational Nursing from UNINTER. Postgraduate student in Culture, Education and Indigenous Health at the INOVA Postgraduate Institute. Nurse at the Special Secretariat for Indigenous Health - SESAI/MS. E-mail: dany.me@hotmail.com

5. Dione Scarabelot Gomes

Nurse, graduated from Faculdade das Américas, 2009. Specialist in Urgency and Emergency Nursing Care UDC, 2013. Specialist in Public Health with an emphasis on Family Health UNINTER 2015. Specialist in Occupational Nursing, UNINTER 2016. Specialist in Indigenous Health and Education at the INOVA Institute. Nurse at the Special Secretariat for Indigenous Health, SESAI/MS.

6. Eduardo Ferraz Ribeiro do Valle Neto

Dentist, graduated from the Julio de Mesquita Filho State University, Faculty of Dentistry of Araçatuba - SP (FOA - UNESP);

Specialist in Indigenous Health, Education and Culture at the INOVA Institute; Dentist at the Special Secretariat for Indigenous Health - SESAI/MS

7. Evaldo Silva do Nascimento

Graduated in Nursing from the Campos Gerais Higher Education Center (CESCAGE), 2004. Specialist in Family Health in Primary Care from the Institute for Postgraduate Studies and Extension (IBPEX), 2007. Specialist in Indigenous Health Education and Culture, 2016. Currently working as a RT nurse at the Special Secretariat for Indigenous Health SESAI/MS. Unidade Bàsica de Saùde Faxinal - E-mail: nascimentoevaldo@hotmail.com

8. Kely Barboza Ribeiro

Dentist, graduated from the State University of Maringà - UEM, 2009. Specialist in Indigenous Health, Education and Culture at Instituto Inova 2016. She is currently responsible for oral health at the DISTRITO SANITARIO ESPECIAL INDIGENA LITORAL SUL - DSEI LSUL/ Secretaria Especial de Saùde Indigena SESAI/MS. E-mail: kelybribeiro@hotmail.com

9. Luzemar das Graças Borges

Nurse. Graduated in nursing from Guairacà College. Specialist in Urgency and Emergency from pre-hospital to ICU at Guairacà College. Specialist in Mental Health and Family Health at UNINTER and Specialist in Health, Education and Indigenous Culture at the INOVA Institute. Nurse at the Municipal Health Department of Candói - Paranà. E-mail: luzemar borges @hotmail.com

10. Paula Regina Jensen

Nurse, graduated from Universidade Estadual do Centro Oeste - UNICENTRO in 2009. Specialist in Public Health at UNOPAR. Specialist in Health Surveillance at UNINTER. Specialist in Indigenous Health, Education and Culture at the INOVA Postgraduate Institute. Nurse at the Special Secretariat for Indigenous Health - SESAI/MS.

11. Rafael de Paula Marcondes

Dental surgeon, graduated from the University of Northern Paranà - UNOPAR, in 2011. Postgraduate in Implant Dentistry from UNOPAR - 2014. Postgraduate degree in Health, Education and Indigenous Culture from the INOVA Institute - 2016. Dental surgeon at the Special Secretariat for Health

Indigenous - SESAI/MS. E-mail: rafaelsoco@hotmail.com

12. Raisa Ottano Peixoto

Nurse, graduated in nursing from the University of Grande Dourados-UNIGRAN in 2012. Specialist in education, health and indigenous culture at the Inova Institute. Nurse at the Special Secretariat for Indigenous Health - SESAI/MS. E-mail: raisaottano@gmail.com

13. Simone Aparecida da Silva

Nurse, graduated from Universidade Paranaense - UNIPAR, 2013, specialist in Urgency and Emergency from UNIPAR, specialist in Indigenous Health, Education and Culture from Instituto INOVA. Nurse at the Special Secretariat for Indigenous Health - SESAI/MS. E-mail: Si mone23@hotmail.com

14. Veronica Tereza Cardoso Zàrrete

Dentist, graduated from the University of the Sacred Heart, 2005. Specialist in Orthodontics at FACOP in 2013. Specialist in Indigenous Health, Education and Culture at the INOVA Institute in 2016. E-mail: vezarete.almeida@hotmail.com

PREFACE

First of all, I congratulate Professor *Clovis Giacomet* for his brilliant initiative as the organizer of this book, and for sharing knowledge about the health, education and culture of Brazil's indigenous peoples. This book has the ability to add value to the training of health professionals who are currently working and those who may yet have the great opportunity to develop their work activities with mastery after reading this book.

The issues surrounding the health policies of indigenous communities have always been delicate, due to a number of factors, including the fact that they live in remote areas that are difficult to access, and as a result they suffer from a number of illnesses, including respiratory infections, hepatitis, sexually transmitted diseases, tuberculosis and others. The texts in this book take us in another worrying direction: the consequences of changes in eating habits, which lead to cultural alterations and highlight the experiences of health and education professionals with these peoples.

It is worth pointing out that before the Brazilian state came into power in 1990 with the Indigenous Protection Service (SPI), and in 1967 with the National Indian Foundation (FUNAI), all the communities used natural products in their diet, making them more resistant to the aforementioned diseases. Since the discovery of Brazil in 1500, when the national indigenous population was estimated at 6 million people, to the present day, where the population is 893,000 citizens (IBGE, 2010), several factors have contributed to the reduction of this population, such as: colonization with slavery, murders, diseases, cultural and dietary changes. By way of illustration, according to the IBGE, one third of the indigenous population works or lives in urban areas.

In one of the works in this book, the structuring of a differentiated care model was brilliantly highlighted, under the responsibility of the Special Indigenous Health Districts - SESAI/MS, mainly since the 1988 Constitution of the Republic and the countless Health Conferences for Indigenous Peoples, which have been taking place in Brazil since 1986.

Among the studies described, the oral health of indigenous people stands out, which has been drastically damaged by dietary changes, such as the introduction of table salt - sodium chloride, sugar and edible oil, as well as other industrialized products, In this context, the role of the professional dentist stands out, who needs to develop and maintain permanent actions in these communities, taking into account the culture of each community spread across this continental country.

Considering the insertion of indigenous people in urban work and the search for education in an environment that is adverse to their own, I am concerned about the social and cultural vulnerability that permeates them, such as financial hyposufficiency, insecurity of housing in peripheries or slums, unemployment, even with the advent of Decree No. 5,051 of April 19, 2004, which promulgated Convention No. 169 of the International Labor Organization (ILO) on indigenous peoples.

Finally, what becomes clear in this work, in the light of the authors' experiences, is the need for differentiated care, whether by the Unified Health System/SUS, or by all other state bodies, when we must consider and respect indigenous people in their social organization, customs, languages, beliefs and traditions.

As a professional in the field of women's health for three decades, I would like to highlight the importance of comprehensive care for indigenous women, especially in their reproductive cycle, because for their people, as I have learned from the indigenous people, population growth is of fundamental importance in order to give continuity to their ancestors, a situation of honor for their community. We have noticed that prenatal care is still weak in terms of quality; it is deficient in terms of uterine cancer control and I would also highlight the weakness in terms of promoting and preventing sexually transmitted infections and others.

In conclusion, you could spend hours writing about this subject, because it is a thought-provoking, contemporary work that is advisable for all professionals in all areas, especially colleagues in health, education and all those human beings who are sensitive to the indigenous cause of our country and the world. And it's good that everyone has them as an example of resistance in maintaining some customs, traditions that have gone through the whole process of civilization.

Nely Dayse Santos da Mata
Doctor of Science

PRESENTATION

The development of the Specialization Course in Indigenous Health, Education and Culture was born out of the need to improve the training of health professionals to work in intercultural environments, with a view to improving health care for indigenous populations by offering quality health education. Indigenous health, configured as an affirmative policy that takes into account the ethnic and cultural specificities of the country's indigenous peoples, became part of the Unified Health System (SUS) in 1999, when the organization of the Special Indigenous Health Districts (DSEI) began, which cater for a complex socio-cultural universe. Indigenous people are present in 80.5% of Brazilian municipalities. According to IBGE (2010), there are 896,971 people, who make up an enormous socio-diversity that is currently expressed in the form of 238 peoples and 180 different languages.

With the implementation of the National Policy for the Health Care of Indigenous Peoples in 2002, there has been a significant increase in the number of health professionals working to care for indigenous populations, both in the villages and in outpatient and hospital services.

From this perspective of multi-professional qualification and the sharing of interdisciplinary experiences, the students of the course had as a proposal for their CBT (Course Conclusion Work), to put down on paper the knowledge they had experienced on the spot in their daily practices and from their learning during the course. With the aim of expressing all the production of Health, Education and Culture of these peoples, this work was conceived, because as an educator and promoter of these professionals we need to make all this material known.

Clovis Luciano Giacomet (Org.)

1. CHANGES IN THE FOOD HABITS OF INDIGENOUS PEOPLE AND THEIR IMPLICATIONS IN THE HEALTH PROCESS.

Andrea do Rocio Schnaider; Clóvis Luciano Giacomet

INTRODUCTION

Indigenous peoples are exposed to environmental and socio-economic transformations, which place them in a highly vulnerable situation with regard to food and nutritional problems. In view of this situation, and because I have been working with the indigenous population for five years, following their health and disease process in relation to their nutritional conditions and lifestyle, this study aims to identify the influences of the indigenous dietary transition and its implications for the health and disease process of the Brazilian indigenous population by means of a literature review.

This is why new epidemiological studies are needed, as well as the standardization of surveys and an efficient and continuous source of data, so that they can be compared in order to find out the real health conditions of indigenous peoples for planning promotion and prevention actions to help control diseases.

Studies have drawn attention to the greater susceptibility to chronic diseases in groups subjected to the modernization of their lifestyle - changes in diet, stress, sedentary lifestyles and obesity, heredity and socio-economic changes have all been considered contributing factors.

In recent years, there has been an increase in the number of indigenous people suffering from hypertension, obesity, nutritional deficiencies and tooth decay, all of which are linked to diet and lifestyle.

So we asked ourselves: what are the implications for the health process of changes in indigenous eating habits? What is health? What is indigenous food like? What healthy eating habits preserve and improve the quality of life of indigenous people?

Based on the World Health Organization's concept of health, in which health is a state of complete physical, mental and social well-being and not merely the absence of disease, and taking into account that complete well-being varies considerably according to individual, temporal and spatial characteristics, health is understood as the ability to relate to the culture and environment in which one belongs. Good health is associated with an increased quality of life. It is well known that a balanced diet, regular physical exercise and emotional well-being are determining factors for a balanced state of health.

The indigenous people's traditional diet was based on corn and manioc, sweet potatoes, pumpkin, beans, peanuts, hunting and fishing. Today, the menu has changed: the school meals themselves, the food basket provided by FUNAI, contains powdered milk, juices, mate tea, chocolate milk, rice, beans, macaroni, cookies and canned goods, a basically industrialized diet that is alien to the culture of these people, and incorporates Western foods into the daily lives of indigenous children, without taking into account the ethnic and cultural differences of the indigenous people. There are several contextual factors that influence indigenous living conditions and their health conditions, an example of which is the process of sedentarization, followed by a diet based on industrialized products, the abandonment of traditional gardens and practices of gathering, hunting and fishing, promoting sharp and very rapid distortions in the way of life and contributing to the emergence of health problems such as hypertension, cholesterol, diabetes, dental caries and deficiency diseases, This is why it is necessary to work in this area in order to visualize the damage caused and act as professionals with health promotion and prevention actions, preserving the culture of these people, encouraging the production of gardens or even community gardens, the school serving food from the indigenous culture in lunch, and encouraging cultural habits such as fishing, hunting and swimming, dancing and the production of handicrafts in order to preserve and maintain the culture of these people.

The aim is to understand the implications of eating habits in the health and disease process of indigenous people. Specific objectives include: defining health; identifying the eating habits of indigenous people; highlighting the importance of changing healthy eating habits in order to preserve and improve the health of the indigenous population.

CHANGES IN INDIGENOUS EATING HABITS

Some studies have drawn attention to the greater susceptibility to chronic diseases in groups subjected to the modernization of their lifestyle, changes in diet, stress, sedentary lifestyle and obesity, heredity and socio-economic changes have been considered contributing factors to this situation (COIMBRA, MATTOS AND KOIFMAM, 2001).

Based on the concept of health of the World Health Organization - WHO, in which health is a state of complete physical, mental and social well-being and not merely the absence of disease, and taking into account that complete well-being varies considerably according to individual, temporal and spatial characteristics, health is understood as the ability to relate to the culture and environment in which one belongs. (OLIVEIRA, et AL 2014)

An individual's health can be determined by his or her own biology, the physical, social and economic environment to which he or she is exposed and his or her lifestyle, i.e. eating habits and other behaviors that can be beneficial or harmful.

Good health is associated with an increased quality of life. It is well known that a balanced diet, regular physical exercise and emotional well-being are determining factors for a balanced state of health.

One of the axes of Brazil's National Health Promotion Policy is healthy eating, which is a human right, having nutritious and adequate food is a basic requirement for quality of life, reducing health risks and seeking comprehensive care (BRASIL, 2008).

Cardoso, Mattos and Koifmam (2001), carried out a study of the prevalence of risk factors in the adult population of the Sapukai, Paraty-Mirim and Arapongas indigenous villages in Rio de Janeiro, after the census the population had its data collected through interviews and clinical and biochemical evaluations, the prevalence in all the samples was respectively for arterial hypertension (4. 8%, 2. 6%, and 7. 4%) and obesity (4. 8%, 3. 6%, and 5. 8%),8%, 2.6%, and 7.4%), overweight (2.6%, 19.5%, and 34.8%), obesity (4.8%, 3.9%, and 5.8%), and lipid changes in total cholesterol (2.8%, 2.7%, and 2.9%) and triglycerides (12.6%, 9.5%, and 15.9%). The results suggest that the population evaluated is at intermediate risk for chronic diseases, showing that efforts should be made to control risk factors.

Auzani and Gordani (2008) researched the Guarani Mbya in Piraquara, Paranà, and reported that the food and nutritional insecurity experienced by these peoples causes complications in their health, such as malnutrition, anemia, hypovitaminosis and tooth decay.

The unfavorable living conditions with environmental and cultural changes, disputes over territories, occupation of land unsuitable for farming, fruit gathering, hunting and fishing result in difficulties for the indigenous people in maintaining their way of being, their religion and their food consumption.

The Indians' traditional diet is based on corn and manioc, but also includes sweet potatoes, pumpkin, beans and peanuts. The school lunch menu doesn't take into account the ethnic and cultural differences of the indigenous people. The village lunch contains powdered milk, juices, mate tea, chocolate milk, rice, beans, macaroni, cookies and canned goods, a basically industrialized diet that is alien to the culture of these people, and incorporates Western foods into the daily lives of indigenous children.

Anemia is a serious nutritional problem in indigenous populations, especially affecting children and women of reproductive age. In addition to insufficient intake of certain nutrients, such as iron, the occurrence of anemia in indigenous populations is probably also associated with the presence of endemic parasites, such as hookworm disease and malaria, according to the study, since most of the work is carried out in the Amazon region.

In the 1960s and 1970s, surveys pointed to high frequencies of anemia among the Xavante (Neel et al., 1964) and in the populations of the Upper Xingu (FAGUNDES NETO, 1977). More recent research has also found that this nutritional deficiency is widespread. Among the Tupi-Mondé, for example, around 60% of children aged 0.5-10 years and 65% of the general population were anemic (SANTOS, 1993). Among the Xavante, Leite (1998) reported the occurrence of anemia in 74% of children aged 0-10 and in 53% of the total population. In the states of Rio de Janeiro and São Paulo, Serafim (1997) detected 69% anemia in Guarani children aged 0-65 months, reaching 82% in those aged 6-24 months.

As for other nutritional deficiencies, it is worth drawing attention to the report by Vieira Filho et al. (1977) about the occurrence of beriberi among the Xavante, which these authors associated with a diet based almost exclusively on processed rice. This record is particularly important, as it points to the serious nutritional impacts that can result from changes in the diet of indigenous groups due to a reduction in dietary diversity.

Speaking of the changes in the Xavantes' diet, this people experienced a decrease over time in their mobility in exploiting the environment, which led to a decrease in hunting and gathering activities and an increase in the importance of agriculture, they became sedentary and there were dietary changes including dependence on industrialized products, their diet based on fruit gathering, hunting became based on rice. (ARANTES; SANTOS and FRAZÂO, 2010)

The case of the Xavante from the village of Eténitepa (or Pimentel Barbosa), in Mato Grosso, illustrates this process well. In the early 1960s, the Xavante were studied by a team of doctors and anthropologists (Neel et al., 1964).

Some 30 years later, the same group was re-studied and the results clearly showed a tendency for systolic and diastolic blood pressure levels to rise.

In 1962, systolic and diastolic pressures were in the range of 94 - 126, 48 - 80 mmHg, respectively, and no cases of hypertension were observed. In 1990, the systolic and diastolic averages were higher in both sexes and cases of hypertension were detected. Also in 1990, there was a positive correlation between systolic blood pressure and age, which had not previously been seen.

Coimbra Jr. and associates argue that over the course of almost 50 years of contact with national society, changes in lifestyle have predisposed the Xavantes to hypertension and other cardiovascular diseases. For example, there has been a significant increase in the average body mass index (BMI) of adults, as well as a reduction in physical activity (SANTOS et al., 1997; GUELMIM & SANTOS, 2001).

Today, rice forms the basis of the diet and salt is used daily. In addition, a significant proportion of indigenous people smoke, which was not the case in the past.

Obesity is a growing health problem among indigenous peoples in the most diverse regions of the world, particularly in North America, Oceania and Polynesia (COIMBRA Jr, SANTOS AND ESCOBAR, 2005).

In relation to indigenous peoples in Brazil, references to the occurrence of obesity are uncommon. With regard to nutritional problems, reviews on the nutritional status of indigenous populations published up until the early 1990s mainly emphasized the occurrence of chronic protein-energy malnutrition and its effects on the physical growth of children (SANTOS, 1993).

Two illustrative cases of the interrelationships between socio-economic and environmental changes and their influence on the nutritional status and body composition of adults are those of the Surui (Santos & Coimbra Jr., 1996) and the Xavante (GUGELMIM E SANTOS, 2001).

At the end of the 1980s, an anthropometric survey of Surui adults showed that those individuals who were no longer directly involved in "traditional" subsistence activities consumed a diet that combined industrialized foods that were low in fibre, high in fat and/or sugar and also had lower levels of physical activity.

These individuals had much higher average weights than the Surui adult population in general. The differences reached 7.6 kg among women and 5.7 kg among men. The authors concluded that the segment of the Surui population that gained the most weight was the one most directly involved in certain newly introduced economic activities, which led to rapid capitalization (through coffee cultivation and the timber trade), causing important changes in diet and patterns of physical activity.

Gugelmin & Santos (2001) compared two Xavante communities with different trajectories of contact and changes in their subsistence systems. They found significantly higher weight and BMI averages in the community where the changes were more intense.

With regard to the nutritional status of mothers, obesity exceeds malnutrition, demonstrating the replacement of the problem of food shortage by excess and inadequate diet among adults. The prevalence of maternal obesity observed in this study (9.2%) is similar to the prevalence in the adult Brazilian population (9.6%) in 1989 (MONTEIRO et al., 2000).

With regard to the qualitative assessment of the diet, the results indicate monotony and inadequacy, where food consumption was determined by insufficient local production and low disposable income, with the purchase of low-quality and lower-cost products. The coexistence of nutritional deficiencies and inadequacies in the composition of the diet was observed, with a high frequency of foods rich in fat and sugar and a low frequency of milk and dairy products, fruit and vegetables. The permanent contact with urban communities surrounding the villages and the marketing of the food industry promotes the accelerated introduction of numerous industrialized products of reduced quality to the detriment of traditional foods (RIBAS, PHILIPPI, 2001).

A healthy diet throughout life contributes to reducing the prevalence of food-related diseases such as obesity, diabetes, heart disease, cancer and tooth decay. Healthy food needs to have some basic attributes such as color, variety, taste, physical and financial accessibility, harmony and food safety. It should reach people from childhood onwards, encouraging healthy habits and respecting people's cultural and food identity (BRASIL, 2008).

Studies of indigenous populations have shown an increase in

cardiovascular diseases, diabetes and mental disorders due to the process of cultural identity crisis and changes in habits, especially eating habits.

Although behavioral changes and cases of chronic diseases have been detected more and more frequently in these populations after contact with the non-indigenous population, it is still common for an epidemiological pattern consisting of infectious diseases and deprivation to coexist (LEITE, 1998).

Even though there are still indigenous societies that maintain a traditional way of life, in which adequate food in quantity and quality comes from hunting and farming, the majority of Indians in Brazil do not have enough land to guarantee their subsistence, mainly due to internal political and economic issues, degradation of the ecosystem - with little native forest, and a lot of land leased to agro-industry.

In addition to abandoning traditional farming practices, which in the past contributed to the diversity of the food consumed, indigenous peoples are exposed to socio-economic transformations, which puts them in a highly vulnerable situation when it comes to food, nutrition and oral health problems (MOURA, BATISTA, MOREIRA, 2010).

For the same author, contact with urban civilization led this population to consume "white people's food" - industrialized food - and to a reduction in physical activity, since what was once obtained through hunting, fishing and subsistence farming - planting corn, manioc, bananas, peanuts, sugar cane, sweet potatoes, pineapples and collecting honey - was now acquired through paid work in urban centers or by producing and selling handicrafts. An example of this cultural transition was observed among the Xavante of Mato Grosso, with a drop in the consumption of cultivated foods and an increase in industrialized foods - sugar, coffee, cooking oil, wheat flour, salt, bread, cookies, powdered soft drinks, soft drinks and candies.

Health care for indigenous peoples is a difficult task for the Brazilian state, due to their social, political and cultural organization and difficulties of access. Indigenous people receive health care through the Indigenous Health Care Subsystem, which is part of the Unified Health System (SUS). The Special Secretariat for Indigenous Health (SESAI) was created by Decree No. 7336 of 19/10/2010 to manage the subsystem throughout the country (BRASIL 2011; BERTANHA, 2012).

The mission of the Special Secretariat for Indigenous Health is to manage, protect, promote and recover the health of indigenous peoples, respecting the policies and programs of the health system, not forgetting the specificities and epidemiological profile of each of the 34 Special Indigenous Health Districts (DSEI). The care provided to indigenous peoples is based on respect for their traditions and their social and cultural diversity (BERTANHA, 2012).

In view of this situation, and because I have been working with the indigenous population for five years and have followed their health and disease process in relation to their nutritional conditions and lifestyle, this study aims to identify the influence of the indigenous dietary transition and its implications for the health-disease process of the Brazilian indigenous population by means of a literature review, which is relevant to the development of actions to prevent and promote indigenous health.

CONCLUSION

By analyzing the various epidemiological works and studies aimed at analyzing changes in indigenous people's eating habits and their determinants, we can see that changes in economic and social patterns interfere in the population's mortality and morbidity profiles, having an effect on infectious diseases as well as chronic non-communicable diseases.

In line with the epidemiological and demographic transition, changes are occurring in the dietary and nutritional patterns of indigenous populations, revealing the complexity of consumption models and their determining factors, where nutritional deficits and obesity coexist, marked by changes in levels of physical activity and the composition of the indigenous diet. The various studies analyzed also point to a picture whose determinants are linked to ecological, socio-economic and health conditions resulting from rapid population growth, environmental degradation, lack of sanitation and difficulty in sustaining food.

It is worth mentioning that even three years after the districtization process began, the SIASI still does not provide comprehensive demographic and epidemiological data. It is hoped that this situation will soon be reversed and that in-depth analyses will begin to monitor and evaluate the health conditions of indigenous peoples under the new health care policy. This will contribute to the existence of systematic epidemiological records which will be of great value for planning, implementing and evaluating health services and programs.

With regard to the qualitative assessment of the diet, the results indicate monotony and inadequacy, where food consumption was determined by insufficient local production and low disposable income, with the purchase of low quality and lower cost products. The coexistence of nutritional deficiencies and inadequacies in the composition of the diet was observed, with a high frequency of industrialized foods. Permanent contact with the urban communities surrounding the villages promotes the accelerated introduction of numerous industrialized products of reduced quality to the detriment of traditional foods.

Guaranteeing quality food for indigenous families depends on access to land and agricultural resources, in order to provide sufficient domestic production, improving the quantitative and qualitative aspects of the diet.

It is necessary to develop educational activities which should include the valorization of traditional foods and cultural activities.

The implementation of measures and improvements in living conditions in these communities depends heavily on the actions of the public sector, i.e. through effective policies and specific investments, mitigating the damaging effects of social inequality.

REFERENCES

AUZANI, SCS; GIORDANI, RCF **Interrelations between physical space, the Mbya- Guarani way of life and food from the perspective of food security:** Reflections on the Araça-I indigenous area in Piraquara/Pr; Espaço Amerindio, Porto Alegre. v.2, n.1. p.129-165 jan/jun 2008.

MOURA, P. G; BATISTA, L. R; MOREIRA, E. A. **Populaçâo Indigena uma reflexâo sobre a Influência da civilização urbana no estado nutricional e na saù.** Campinas: Rev. de Nutriçâo, 23(3) 459-465, May/Jun, 2010.

ARANTES, R; SANTOS, RV; COIMBRA JR, CEA. **Oral health in the Xavante indigenous population of Pimentel Barbosa in Mato Grosso, Brazil.** Cad. Saùde Pùblica. Rio de Janeiro: v.17, n.2, p. 375-384, May/April, 2001.

CARDOSO, A. M; MATTOS, I. E; KOIFMAM, R. J. **Prevalência de fatores de risco para doenças cardiovasculares na populaçâo Guarani- Mbya do estado do Rio d Janeiro**. Rio de Janeiro: Caderno de Saùde Pùblica, 17(2); 345- 354, March and April 2001.

BRAZIL. Ministry of Health. Secretariat of Health Care. **Operational manual for health and education professionals.** Promoting healthy eating in schools, 2008. Brasilia, 152p.

BERTANHA, W.F.F. et al. Oral Health Care in Indigenous Communities:

Evolution and Challenges - A Literature Review. **Brazilian Journal of Health** Sciences-v 16, n 1:105-112, 2012.

LEONARDO, M. **Anthropology of Food**. Rev. Artigos, vol. 3. ano 2, dez 2009-ISSN-1982-1050.

BRAZIL. Ministry of Health. Health Care Secretariat. **Guidelines for the National Indigenous Oral Health Policy** (preliminary version). Brasilia, 2011.12 p.

COIMBRA JR., CEA., SANTOS, RV and ESCOBAR, AL., orgs. **Epidemiologia e saùde dos povos indìgenas no Brasil [online]**. Rio de Janeiro: Editora FIOCRUZ; Rio de Janeiro: ABRASCO, 2005. 260 p. ISBN: 85-7541-022-9. ` Available from SciELO Books <http://books.scielo.org>.

COIMBRA Jr., C. E. A. & SANTOS, R. V., 1991. **Evaluation of nutritional status in a context of socio-economic change:** The Surui indigenous group in the state of Rondônia, Brazil. Cadernos de Saùde Pùblica, 7:538-562.

BLOCH, K. V.; COUTINHO, E. S. F.; LÔBO, M. E. C.; OLIVEIRA, J. E. P. & MILECH, A., 1993. **Blood pressure, capillary glycemia and anthropometric measurements in a Yanomami population.** Cadernos de Saùde Pùblica, 9:428-438.

LEITE, M. S., 1998. **Avaliação do Estado Nutricional da Populaçâo Xavante de Sâo José, Terra Indigena Sangradouro - Volta Grande, Mato Grosso.** Master's dissertation, Rio de Janeiro: National School of Public Health, Oswaldo Cruz Foundation.

GUGELMIM, S. A., 1995. **Nutrition and Time Allocation of the Xavantes of Pimentel Barbosa, Mato Grosso:** A Study in Human Ecology and Change. Master's dissertation, Rio de Janeiro: National School of Public Health, Oswaldo Cruz Foundation.

OLIVEIRA, S. P. & THÉBAUD-MONY, A., 1997. **Studying food consumption:** in search of a multidisciplinary approach. Revisto de Saùde Pùblica, 31:201-208

GUGELMIN, S. A. & SANTOS, R. V, 2001. **Human ecology and nutritional anthropometry of Xavante adults, Mato Grosso, Brazil.** Cadernos de Saùde Pùblica, 17:313-322.

ARANTES, R.; SANTOS RV; FRAZAO P. **Differentials of dental caries among the Xavantes Indians of Mato Grosso, Brazil.** Rev. Bras. Epidemiologia. v.13, n.2, p. 223-236, 2010.

CARDOSO, A. M.; MATTOS, I. E. & KOIFMAN, R. J., 2 0 0 1. **Prevalence of risk factors for cardiovascular diseases in the Guarani-Mbyà population of the State of Rio de Janeiro.** Cadernos de Saùde Pùblica, 17:345-354.

SANTOS, R. V., 1993. **Physical growth and nutritional status of Brazilian indigenous populations.** Cadernos de Saùde Pùblica, 9 (Suppl. 1):46-57.

RIBAS, D. L. B., 2001. **Health and Nutrition of Teréna Indigenous Children, Mato Grosso do Sul, Brazil.** PhD Thesis, Sao Paulo: School of Public Health, University of Sao Paulo.

MONTEIRO, C. A.; BENiCIO, M. H. A.; GOUVEIA, N. C. & CARDOSO, M. A. A.,2000. Evolution of child malnutrition. In: **Velhos e Novos Males da Saùde no Brasil** (C. A. Monteiro, org.), pp. 93-114, Sao Paulo: Hucitec.

FAGUNDES-NEÏO, U., 1977. **Evaluation of the Nutritional Status of Indian Children of the Upper Xingu.** Doctoral thesis, Sao Paulo: Escola Paulista de Medicina.

SERAFIM, M. G., 1997. **Eating Habits and Hemoglobin Levels in Indigenous Children.** Guarani, Under 5 Years of Age, from the States of Sao Paulo and Rio de Janeiro. Master's dissertation, Sao Paulo: Paulista School of Medicine.

VIEIRA FILHO. P. B., 1977. Diabetes mellitus and the fasting glucose levels of the Caripuna and

Palikur. **Revista da Associaçâo Mèdica Brasileira**, 23:175-178.

SANTOS, R. V., 1993. **Physical growth and nutritional status of Brazilian indigenous populations.** Cadernos de Saùde Pùblica, 9 (Suppl. 1):46-57.

2. CULTURAL CHANGES RELATED TO HEALTH INSERTED INTO THE INDIGENOUS COMMUNITY THROUGH COEXISTENCE WITH NON-INDIGENOUS SOCIETIES

Daiza Martins Lopes Goncalves, Clóvis Luciano Giacomet

INTRODUCTION

According to data from the Demographic Census carried out by the IBGE - Brazilian Statute of Geography and Statistics, in 2010, the indigenous population in Brazil numbered approximately 869,900, distributed among 305 ethnic groups, the largest of which was the Tikùna, speaking 274 languages. According to the census, 37.4% of indigenous people aged 5 and over spoke an indigenous language and 76.9% spoke Portuguese (BRASIL, 2015).

These indigenous peoples are distributed throughout Brazil's five regions, with the North having the largest number of individuals and the South the smallest. Of the total number of indigenous people, 63.8% live in rural areas and 36.2% live in urban areas. Throughout Brazil, 505 indigenous lands have been demarcated, which represents only 12.5% of the Brazilian territory (BRASIL, 2015).

This data shows how the indigenous people have suffered a reduction in their population, since before colonization there were an estimated 5 million Indians spread across the territory, according to Fausto (1996).

This reduction in population was mainly due to the process of enslavement suffered during Portuguese and Spanish colonization, at the end of the 15th century and throughout the 16th century, with the discovery of America and the taking of possession of the newly discovered lands (FAUSTO, 1996).

Since then, the indigenous people have been subjected to a process of acculturation which, according to Rodrigues (2014), is due to the contact between different cultures and the mutual adoption of customs belonging to the different culture.

Before the arrival of the Portuguese, the indigenous people had a socially, culturally and religiously structured way of life. This structure was directly influenced by the colonizers, causing many customs to be set aside, both by imposition and by the very will of the indigenous people who "got used to" some of the non-indigenous ways of life (FAUSTO, 1996).

Among the aspects that were influenced by colonization was the way in which indigenous people perceive the health-disease process and how the diseases brought by non-indigenous people contributed to the reduction in the indigenous population already described here.

Since the researcher works in an indigenous health unit and is able to observe this context, these issues raised the desire to delve deeper into the subject, justifying the present study, which aims to verify how the cultural changes introduced into indigenous populations by living with non-indigenous populations have affected their perception of the health-disease process.

INDIGENOUS PEOPLE IN BRAZIL

The history of the Brazilian Indians began with the accounts of Pero Vaz de Caminha when the expedition arrived in Brazil.

of Pedro Alvares Cabral to Brazil who, according to history, got lost on the way to the Indies, on the Asian continent in search of gold, precious stones and spices.

This was the beginning of the decimation of a people who, before the arrival of the non-Indians, lived in an organized and structured society, divided into tribes according to the region in which they lived. Each tribe had its own way of life, where the men were generally responsible for hunting, fishing and making tools for these purposes and the women and children for gathering fruit and seeds, making tools and maintaining the huts. There was also a clear hierarchy to be respected, in the form of chiefs, shamans and elders who were extremely respected.

Their customs and beliefs were based on elements of nature and they worshipped these elements as gods, namely the sun, rain, thunder, etc.

They also fought for territory and defended their tribe from others and from animals that might pose a threat. Their illnesses were cured by the shaman, the tribe's healer, using herbs and roots. Until then, not many diseases affecting non-Indians from civilized continents were known.

However, as nothing of "value" had been discovered in Brazil, despite being declared a colony of Portugal, it remained abandoned for almost thirty years, with only brazilwood, a wood of good commercial value in Europe, being harvested from here. With the intention of protecting the colony, the king of Portugal decided to colonize Brazil through the system of hereditary captaincies, donating the land divided into 15 parts distributed to 12 grantees and thus marking the beginning of the enslavement and sublimation of the indigenous peoples who lived in Brazilian territory.

Realizing that the indigenous people were docile and easily manipulated, they began to be used as labour in the sesmarias, being treated inhumanely, because, for the Portuguese, they didn't have souls and therefore didn't deserve any humane treatment.

Fausto (1996) states that the enslavement of the Indian came up against a series of drawbacks, in view of the aims of colonization. The Indians had a culture that was incompatible with intensive and regular labor, and even more so with enslavement, as the Europeans intended. They were not idle or lazy. They only did what was necessary to guarantee their subsistence, which wasn't difficult at a time of abundant fish, fruit and animals.

Much of their energy and imagination was employed in rituals, celebrations and warfare. The notions of continuous work or what today would be called productivity were totally foreign to them.

There were two basic attempts by the Portuguese to enslave the Indians. One of them, carried out by the settlers according to a cold economic calculation, consisted of pure and simple enslavement. The other was attempted by the religious orders, especially the Jesuits, for reasons that had a lot to do with their missionary conceptions. It consisted of the effort to transform the Indians, through teaching, into "good Christians", bringing them together in small towns or villages. Being a "good Christian" also meant acquiring the work habits of Europeans, which would create a group of indigenous cultivators who were flexible to the needs of the colony.

However, the intentions of these different groups were opposed. The religious orders had the merit of trying to protect the Indians from the slavery imposed by the settlers, which led to a lot of friction between settlers and priests. But the priests also had no respect for indigenous culture. On the contrary, for them it was even doubtful that the Indians were people, as mentioned above. "Father Manuel da Nóbrega, for example, said that 'Indians are dogs when it comes to eating and killing, and pigs when it comes to vices and the way they treat each other'" (FAUSTO, 1996).

Thus, the Indians who were subjected to enslavement gradually lost their customs and beliefs and obeyed the customs of the non-whites, even praying in Latin.

With contact with the non-Indians, in addition to the process of acculturation, also came diseases such as measles, variola, influenza, against which the Indians had no resistance, decimating thousands of them, according to Fausto, 1996):

Two epidemic waves stood out for their violence between 1562 and 1563, killing more than 60,000 Indians, it seems, not counting the victims in the hinterland. The death of the indigenous population, which was partly dedicated to planting food crops, resulted in a terrible famine in the Northeast and a loss of arms.

The loss of the Indians then led to the arrival of black slaves in Brazil, a practice that was already well advanced in Europe and which eased the situation of indigenous slavery in Brazil, but did not make them free or give them back their way of life.

Since then, the indigenous population, who were "the owners of the land", have lived on the margins of society.

According to the National Indian Foundation - FUNAI, there are more than 800,000 Indians living in Brazil today, around 0.4% of the Brazilian population, according to data from the 2010 Census. They are distributed among 505 Indigenous Lands and some urban areas. There are also 77 references to uncontacted indigenous groups, 30 of which have been confirmed. There are also groups that are applying for recognition of their indigenous status from the federal indigenist body.

The process of acculturation undergone by the indigenous people in Brazil has left its mark, which is now a cause of concern for movements linked to the indigenous people, especially with regard to health, since many "problems" exclusive to non-indigenous people frighteningly affect the indigenous populations, such as alcoholism and suicide among them, which is growing every day.

THE PROCESS OF ACCULTURATION

According to Ribeiro (2015), the process of acculturation takes place when two or more distinct cultural matrices come into contact through social interaction between groups from different cultures and when all or one of them undergoes changes, resulting in a new culture, but this new culture will be based on elements of its initial cultural matrices.

Laraia (2008) says It is possible to state that acculturation would be a form of cultural transformation promoted by external factors (contact between diverse cultural patterns) - opposed to that permanent process that occurs within the culture itself, that is, within the society itself throughout history. It is important to say that the values and customs of a given people can change according to the 'dynamics of the cultural system itself'.

Thus, in the author's view, the process of acculturation can take place in various ways, in a milder or more imposing manner, over a long period of time or quickly. However, a relationship of power between groups is always present, as in the case of the colonization of the Americas by the Portuguese and Spanish, where this process of acculturation in relation to the indigenous people was extremely violent and domineering, instilling in them customs and values such as Catholicism imposed as a religion.

However, Laraia (2008) points out that the process of acculturation does not always represent only negative aspects, since the cultural aspects of different ethnicities can be assimilated naturally, citing as an example the immigrants of various nationalities who arrived in Brazil, mainly because of the Second World War and who contributed significantly to the cultural formation of the Brazilian people in various aspects.

As far as the indigenous are concerned, the process of acculturation has taken place since the arrival of the Portuguese in Brazil more than 500 years ago, and the first transformation that took place was in religion. The indigenous people who lived here had their beliefs based on the divinities of nature and Catholicism was imposed on them in a radical way by the Jesuit priests, and they even had to pray in Latin, when they didn't even speak Portuguese (JUNQUEIRA, 1991).

From then on, other aspects of indigenous culture were affected: the language itself, food, clothing and others, which ended up being assimilated by the Indians, either by imposition or by the "comforts" that the new customs provided (JUNQUEIRA, 1991).

The health of indigenous people and the way in which they were cared for also underwent a drastic transformation, since before the arrival of the Portuguese, numerous illnesses were unknown to them, which later became part of the population's routine, such as colds, infections and other comorbidities related to their way of life. What had previously only been treated with herbal remedies and "prayers" began to require more complex treatments to which they did not always have access (JUNQUEIRA, 1991).

UNDERSTANDING THE HEALTH-DISEASE PROCESS

According to Câmara et al. (2012), although various concepts of the health-disease process have been established, over time this concept has been transformed according to the different ways in which society exists, which is constantly changing with the acquisition of new knowledge and the transformation of its culture and forms of organization.

The understanding of both health and illness depends on one's understanding of the relationships established with the environment in which one lives, which can vary according to the place, culture and historical moment in which one lives.

According to Vianna (2012), "illness cannot be understood only by means of pathophysiological measurements, because what establishes the state of illness is suffering, pain, pleasure, in short, the values and feelings expressed by the subjective body that falls ill".

Meanwhile, the World Health Organization defines health as "a state of complete physical, mental and social well-being and not merely the absence of disease and infirmity". Most authors on the subject criticize this definition, since a complete balance between physical, mental and social well-being in the turbulent times in which society currently lives sounds like a utopia (SEGRE; FERRAZ, 1997).

Brêtas and Gamba (2006) consider that:

[...] for health, it is necessary to start from the dimension of being, because it is there that the definitions of normal or pathological occur. What is considered normal in one individual may not be in another; there is no rigidity in the process. In this way, we can deduce that human beings need to know themselves, they need to be able to evaluate the transformations their bodies undergo and identify the signs they express. This process is only possible from a relational perspective, because normal and pathological can only be appreciated in a relationship.

Thus, Vianna (2012) argues that for a more complete view of the health-disease process, it is necessary to take into account the distinction between disease as defined by care systems and health as perceived by individuals, also including the dimension of well-being in a broader sense.

For Brêtas and Gambà (2006):

[...] health and illness are not two sides of the same coin. In fact, if we consider a health system such as the SUS, it is possible to see that actions aimed at diagnosing and treating diseases are only two of its activities. Social inclusion, promoting equity or visibility and citizenship are considered health actions. The understanding of health as a

relatively autonomous social device in relation to the idea of illness, and the repercussions that this new understanding brings to social life and everyday practices in general and health services in particular, opens up new possibilities in the conception of the health and illness process.

As you can see, the understanding of the health-disease process varies according to people's conceptions of the time, culture and region.

UNDERSTANDING THE HEALTH-DISEASE PROCESS

In the research carried out by Silva, Gonçalves and Lopes Neto (2003), in two indigenous villages in Amazonas, with the aim of verifying the indigenous people's understanding of the health-disease process, the authors were able to see that the indigenous people did not understand the seriousness of certain health problems, nor did they establish links between the disease and its causes, which the researchers attributed to a lack of sanitation, hygiene and preventive actions.

Fracolli and Bertolozzi (2001) consider that the understanding of "[...] health/disease is directly linked to the way in which human beings, over the course of their existence, have appropriated nature in order to transform it, seeking to meet their needs".

The indigenous people, despite already having a fairly advanced culture, still have their own beliefs and way of life, making it difficult for them to learn about the disease and its causes, as well as forms of prevention and treatment.

In this sense, Langdon (2000) states that "it is essential to respect the notions, values and expectations of each ethnic group". In this vein, it is important to emphasize that the principle of the National Policy for the Health Care of Indigenous Peoples preaches "[...] respect for the conceptions, values and practices relating to the health/disease process specific to each indigenous society" (BRASIL, 2002).

In a study carried out by Lazarotto and Baratieri, et.al., 2007), it became clear that, of the 132 Kaingang families who took part, the majority based their beliefs about health/disease on their own indigenous culture and that customs and beliefs are also linked to the search for the most important figure in the village, who is the shaman. It is based on his opinion that they seek treatment at the health unit.

Analyzing the results of this research, we can see that, despite having medical assistance, the belief in the shaman's "diagnosis" is still predominant and it is on his advice that they go to seek help at the medical clinic, making it clear that respect for the values of each ethnic group must be taken into account, as advised by the National Policy on Health Care for Indigenous Peoples.

In the research by Pellon and Vargas (2010), carried out in three villages in Espirito Santo, it became clear that the perceptions of indigenous people also take into account the ethnic values of their culture, because, according to these authors: Cultural practice recommends that the illness be diagnosed within the *opy* (prayer house) by the *Karai* (shaman) who should indicate the appropriate treatment, not depriving himself of referring the patient to the public health care system if he deems it necessary.

However, Pellon and Vargas (2007) cite in their research the dissatisfaction of indigenous people with the type of care provided in health units due to the prejudice and ethnocentrism shown by some professionals, which leads them to avoid seeking health care, making it clear that:

[...] the ways in which discrimination is expressed are not always so obvious, because they are often subliminally embedded in the webs of social and economic relationships that structure and determine the expression of the health-disease process, both its direct and indirect

determinants. However, experiencing situations of discrimination can in itself be a trigger for illness and becomes more serious when the experience takes place within health care services, as it can generate strong emotions, ranging from fear and mistrust to anger and frustration, compromising not only the quality and credibility of the services provided, but the individual's own health (PELLON; VARGAS, 2007).

This shows that indigenous people's understanding of the health-disease process is linked to their cultural and ethnic perceptions and values, and that differentiated care for this community is essential because of these peculiarities.

CONCLUSION

The indigenous population in Brazil has been undergoing a process of acculturation since the arrival of the Portuguese, who in one way or another ended up imposing their customs, beliefs and values on the indigenous people, causing many aspects of their culture to be modified.

This process of acculturation takes place gradually and transforms the indigenous people's view of their own culture and, today, the tiny existing population (compared to that at the beginning of colonization) has in many cases lost its references and adopted new ways of life. This can be seen in the alarming numbers of illnesses that were previously not part of indigenous daily life and also in the habits acquired through living with non-indigenous societies, such as the high incidence of alcoholism, for example, which leads to other significant factors such as the high suicide rates among the Indians, especially the younger ones.

When it comes to health, the comorbidities presented are also a cause for concern, despite the fact that the indigenous population receives differentiated health care.

The aim of this study was to see how the cultural changes brought about in indigenous populations by living with non-indigenous populations have affected their perception of the health-disease process, and it was concluded that indigenous people's perception of the health-disease process, despite the process of acculturation they have undergone, they still rely heavily on the knowledge of the tribal elders to cure various ailments, especially those they attribute to "evil spirits", but specialized medical assistance is also widely sought.

REFERENCES

BRAZIL. In Brazil, the indigenous population is 869.9 thousand. **Portal Brasil**. 2015. Available at:

http://www.brasil.gov.br/governo/2015/04/populacao-indigena-no-brasil-e-de-896-9-mil Accessed on 15/01/2016.

BRÊTAS, A. C. P.; GAMBA, M. A. **Enfermagem e saùde do adulto**. Barueri: Manole, 2006.

CÂMARA, A. M. C. S.; MELO, V. L. C.; et.al. Perception of the Health-Disease Process: Meanings and Values of Health Education. **Brazilian Journal of Medical Education.** 2012. Available at: http://www.scielo.br/pdf/rbem/v36n1s1/v36n1s1a06.pdf Accessed on 12/03/2016.

FAUSTO, B. **História do Brasil covers a period of more than five hundred years, from the roots of Portuguese colonization to the present day**. EDUSP. 1996. Available at:

http://www.caccto.com.br/material/d00044/Material 6 EMED 2A 195641.pdf Accessed on 05/01/2016.

FRACOLI, L. A.; BERTOLOZZI, M. R. The approach to the health-disease process of family members and the collective. In: BRASIL. Instituto de

Health Development. University of Sao Paulo. Ministry of Health.

Nursing manual. Brasilia: IDS/USP/MS, 2001.

NATIONAL INDIAN FOUNDATION - FUNAI. **The Indians**. Available at: http://www.funai.gov.br/indios/conteudo.htm Accessed on 10/01/2016.

JUNQUEIRA, C. **Indigenous anthropology**. Sao Paulo: Educ, 1991.

LANGDON, E. J. **Health and Indigenous Peoples**: The challenges at the turn of the century.   1999.   Available at:

http://www.cfh.ufsc.br/~nessi/Margsav.htm Accessed on 15/03/2016.

LARAIA, R. de B. **Cultura**: um conceito antropológico. Rio de Janeiro, Jorge Zahar, 2008.

LAZZAROTTO, E. M.; BARATIERI, T.; et.al. **Existing diseases in the Kaingang and Guarani indigenous community**. 3rd National Seminar on the State and Social Policies in Brazil. UNIOESTE. 2007. Available at: http://www.unioeste.br/prg/prolind/docs/doencas_existentes_comuni dade indigena kaingang guarani.pdf Accessed on 02/03/2016.

PELLON, L. H.; VARGAS, L. A. **Culture, interculturality and the health-disease process:** (dis)paths in health care for the Guarani Mbyà of   Aracruz,   Espirito   Santo.   2007.   Available   at: http://www.scielo.br/scielo.php?pid=S0103-73312010000400017&script=sci arttext Accessed on 09/03/2016.

RIBEIRO, P. S. "What is acculturação all about?"; **Brasil Escola**. Available at: http://brasilescola.uol.com.br/sociologia/do-que-se- trata-aculturacao.htm Accessed on 21/03/2016.

RODRIGUES, L. de O. Aculturação. **Mundo Educação On Line**, 2015.   Available at   at:

http://mundoeducacao.bol.uol.com.br/sociologia/aculturacao.htm Accessed on 15/02/2016.

SEGRE, M.; FERRAZ, F. C. **The concept of health**. 1997. Available at:

http://www.scielo.br/scielo.php?script=sci arttext&pid=S0034-89101997000600016 Accessed on 15/03/2016.

SILVA, N. C. da; GONÇALVES, M. J. F.; LOPES NETO, D. **Enfermagem em saùde indigena**: aplicando as diretrizes curriculares; 2006. Available Available at:

http://www.scielo.br/scielo.php?script=sci arttext&pid=S0034-71672003000400016 Accessed on 06/03/2016.

VIANNA, L. A. C. **Health-disease process**. 2012. Available at: http://www.unasus.unifesp.br/biblioteca virtual/esf/1/modulo politico gestor/Unidade 6.pdf Accessed on: 09/03/2016.

3. NUTRITIONAL STATUS OF INDIGENOUS CHILDREN

Danieli Maria Menon, Clóvis Luciano Giacomet

INTRODUCTION

Brazil's indigenous population was approximately five million at the time of the arrival of the colonizers. Today, according to data from FUNAI - the National Indian Foundation, the indigenous population in Brazil is made up of 490,000 people, belonging to 220 peoples who speak more than 180 languages.

In an effort to provide differentiated care for these populations, since August 1999, the Ministry of Health, through FUNASA - the National Health Foundation, has taken on the responsibility of structuring care for indigenous populations, with the creation of the National Policy for Health Care for Indigenous Peoples, an integral part of the National Health Policy, which provides for the right of these populations to differentiated care by the Unified Health System (SUS), respecting the cultural specificities of each indigenous people (FUNAI, 2013).

The Indigenous Health Subsystem of the Unified Health System (SUS) is organized into 34 Special Indigenous Health Districts - DSEI. It is a dynamic, geographically, populationally and administratively well-defined ethnic-cultural space, which is not directly related to the boundaries of the states and municipalities where the indigenous lands are located (BRASIL, 2002).

Thus, the public authorities, through FUNAI and the Ministry of Health, seek to offer differentiated care to indigenous populations, since the specificities of these peoples require care geared to their conditions, their culture, in short, their way of life.

Brazilian legislation, through Law No. 9.836 of September 23, 1999, art. 19 F, provides for health care, stating that it must be provided to indigenous populations, and that it must "take into account the local reality and the specificities of the culture of indigenous peoples and the model to be adopted for indigenous health care, which must be based on a differentiated and global approach, taking into account the aspects of health care" (BRASIL, 1999), it is necessary to acquire knowledge that can deal with this care in an effective way, and this is what this research project aims to do.

Given that the researcher works directly in an indigenous community as part of the multidisciplinary team that cares for its individuals, observing the nutritional status of indigenous children, there was an interest in delving deeper into the subject in order to improve the care provided, improving the quality of life with regard to their nutritional conditions, thus justifying the present study.

INDIGENOUS HEALTH IN BRAZIL

According to FUNASA (2002), since the beginning of Portuguese colonization, indigenous people were cared for by missionaries in a way that was integrated into government policies. At the beginning of the 20th century, with territorial and economic expansion, which brought with it the construction of railroad and telegraph lines, there were countless massacres of indigenous peoples and a huge rise in mortality rates from communicable diseases, This led to the creation, in 1910, of the Service for the Protection of Indians and National Workers, attached to the Ministry of Agriculture, with the aim of protecting Indians and progressively integrating their lands into the national production system.

However, the indigenous people were still seen as individuals in evolution, considered to be at an infantile stage of humanity and the assistance provided was sporadic and disorganized, limited to emergency or "pacifist" actions. This situation lasted until the 1950s, with no public policies aimed at systematic care, which resulted in many deaths from infectious and contagious diseases affecting the indigenous populations, until the Air Sanitary Units Service was created, which aimed to bring health actions to populations in areas that were difficult to access, essentially focused on vaccination, dental care, tuberculosis control and other communicable diseases (BRASIL, 2002).

In 1967, the Service for the Protection of Indians and National Workers was abolished and FUNAI and the Volante Health Teams were created, which provided sporadic assistance to the indigenous communities in their area of coverage, providing medical care, administering vaccines and supervising the work of the health personnel in these locations, who were limited to nursing assistants and attendants. However, this service fell into decline after the financial crisis that hit Brazil in the 1970s, causing resources for care to become scarce, further compromising the services provided, in addition to the extinction of the Volante Health Teams, which ended up dissolving due to a lack of professionals who ended up settling in urban centers and in administrative activities, returning to a model of emergency and palliative care, provided by people with little qualification.

It is noteworthy that none of the initiatives related to the care of indigenous populations took into account the specificity of this population, ignoring their values, representations and practices related to health and illness, demonstrating disrespect for the context of the indigenous individual's relationship with society and the environment in which they lived.

The situation described only changed with the 1988 Constitution, which "stipulated the recognition and respect of the socio-cultural organizations of indigenous peoples, guaranteeing them full civil capacity - making the institution of guardianship obsolete - and established the exclusive competence of the Union to legislate and deal with indigenous issues"

(BRASIL, 2002, p.8). The Constitution also defined the general principles of the Unified Health System (SUS), later regulated by Law 8.080/90, and established that the sole direction and responsibility for the federal management of the system lies with the Ministry of Health.

Since then, discussions have taken place in order to structure a system capable of offering more effective and timely health care to the indigenous population, as was the case with the First National Conference on the Protection of Indigenous Health and the Second National Conference on Health for Indigenous Peoples, which took place in 1986 and 1993 respectively, on the recommendation of the Eighth and Ninth National Health Conferences.

These two Conferences proposed the structuring of a differentiated model of care, based on the strategy of Special Indigenous Health Districts, as a way of guaranteeing indigenous peoples the right to universal and comprehensive access to health, meeting the needs perceived by the communities and involving the indigenous population in all stages of the process of planning, executing and evaluating actions (BRASIL, 2002).

In 1991, as part of the actions guided by the above-mentioned Conferences, by means of a decree, the government transferred responsibility for coordinating health actions aimed at indigenous populations to the Ministry of Health, establishing the Special Indigenous Health Districts as the basis for organizing health services. The Ministry of Health then created the Coordination of Indigenous Health (COSAI), which was responsible for implementing a new model of indigenous health care (BRASIL, 2002).

In 1997, the Inter-Sectoral Commission on Indigenous Health of the National Health Council (CISI/CNS) requested the intervention of the Federal Public Prosecutor's Office (6- CCR/MPF) because of the federal government's failure to implement an adequate policy for indigenous health care. The public hearing held in November 1997 concluded that the responsibility established in the Federal Constitution for indigenous health care lay with the Ministry of Health at the federal level, and that "the refusal of institutions linked to the SUS to provide this assistance constituted an illegal act that could be confronted through the competent channels" (ALTINI, et.al., 2013).

In view of the serious health problems faced by indigenous peoples, in 1999 the federal government sanctioned Law No. 9.836, adding provisions to Law No. 8.080, of 1990, laying down the conditions for the promotion, protection and recovery of health, the organization and functioning of the corresponding services in relation to indigenous populations, establishing, at that time, the Indigenous Health Care Subsystem, which is linked to the Department of Indigenous Health Care.

According to Ministry of Health Ordinance No. 2607, of December 10, 2004, the Special Indigenous Health Districts are a model for organizing services, which include a set of technical activities, aimed at rationalized and qualified health care measures, promoting the reorganization of the health network and health practices and developing administrative-managerial activities necessary for the provision of care, with social control (BRASIL, 2002).

MALNUTRITION

Malnutrition, according to Chagas, *et.al.* (2013), is characterized as a pathological condition resulting from a lack of energy and protein, in varying proportions, which can be aggravated by repeated infections and, according to Fernandes (2003), is the main alteration of nutritional status because it is one of the main health problems in developing countries, It is estimated that there are currently approximately 800 million chronically malnourished people worldwide, of whom 200 million are moderately or severely malnourished children and 70 million are severely malnourished.

Surui, Mariano and Rios (2014) characterize malnutrition as a state of varying degrees of intensity and varied clinical manifestations produced by the lack of intake of energy-protein foods, as well as: proteins, carbohydrates, fats, mineral salts and vitamins, the lack of which results in the body not being able to assimilate the appropriate amounts of the components needed by the body.

The authors state that:

It comprises a series of diseases, each of which has a specific cause related to a lack of the aforementioned nutrients, and is characterized by the existence of a cellular imbalance between the supply of nutrients and energy on the one hand, and on the other, the body's demand to ensure growth, maintenance and specific functions for the organism. It is an evolutionary deficiency disease, exclusively linked to the age of latency, affecting and altering the function of the growth cell (SURUI, MARIANO, RIOS, 2014).

Jonsson (1986) broadens the concept, making it more comprehensive when he says that malnutrition is "the deterioration in the state of health and productive and social performance of individuals resulting from an intake of food either of poor quality or of the wrong type, or both".

Chagas, *et.al.* (2013) point to evidence that malnutrition in childhood is associated with higher mortality rates, the occurrence of infectious diseases, damage to psychomotor and cognitive development, decreased height and productive capacity. In females, it is associated with a higher risk of having children with low birth weight, demonstrating the intergenerational effect of malnutrition.

Fernandes (2003) points out the main characteristics of child malnutrition, which are as follows:

- It prevails in less developed countries and sectors;

- It affects the most biologically vulnerable individuals, i.e. children under the age of five;

- It is strongly associated with increased morbidity and mortality rates and is one of the most sensitive indicators of a country's social situation.

When it comes to indigenous children, it must be remembered that malnutrition is an aspect that is strongly linked to the values of the community, which has no knowledge of nutritional needs, in addition to the difficulty of obtaining food many times and the poor health conditions in the villages, as well as the inefficiency of public policies in the area of health in the care of indigenous communities.

THE NUTRITIONAL PROFILE OF INDIGENOUS BRAZILIAN CHILDREN

To begin this section, it is interesting to note that Kühl, Corso, Leite and Bastos (2009) cite the scarcity of epidemiological and demographic information on indigenous peoples, which hinders the development of social and health interventions.

In view of this context, the Indigenous Health Care Information System (SIASI) was created in 2000, as part of the National Policy for Indigenous Peoples' Health Care, but it remains partially implemented and presents difficulties and deficiencies with regard to collection instruments and training of human resources, demonstrating that there is still much to be done with regard to a clear mapping of the situation of indigenous health in Brazil (KÜHL; CORSO; LEITE; BASTOS, 2009).

The situation with regard to food and nutritional aspects is no different, but since the 1990s, a growing number of publications have improved the database that can be consulted to outline the nutritional profile of indigenous children (KÜHL; CORSO; LEITE; BASTOS, 2009).

In a study published by UNICEF in 2006, it was found that in 2004 and 2005 there were a significant number of deaths of indigenous children associated with malnutrition in the states of Mato Grosso and Mato Grosso do Sul, involving Guarani-Kaiowàs Indians from the Dourados reserve and Xavante Indians. In the first four months of 2005 alone, there were 21 deaths of children under the age of five in Mato Grosso do Sul and 6 in Mato Grosso, drawing attention to the serious nutritional situation of indigenous children, which, according to UNICEF (2006), has been little considered in the latest national research into child malnutrition.

After explaining this context, an external commission was set up in the Chamber of Deputies to investigate the occurrence of deaths in the states mentioned and it was found that they were not restricted to the cases reported in these years, since between 2003 and 2004 FUNASA had already recorded 32 deaths of indigenous children due to malnutrition in Mato Grosso do Sul and the malnutrition rate was 12%, double the national average (UNICEF, 2006).

However, the death of indigenous children due to malnutrition has also been recorded in the states of Minas Gerais, the northeast of the country, the Javari valley and Amazonas. The alarming situation in Mato Grosso do Sul led to a series of measures being taken to minimize the problem in the state, including the distribution of mega doses of vitamin A by Funasa for children under five, since the lack of vitamin A compromised the children's cognitive and psychomotor development, as well as vision problems, weakening of the immune system, which increases the occurrence of diarrhea and other diseases that can lead to death (UNICEF, 2006).

Another measure taken was to take care of indigenous pregnant women, as a lack of vitamins during pregnancy can lead to miscarriages, malformation of the fetus and premature birth or severe mental retardation. Thus, iodine and folic acid, which are essential for the formation of the baby during the gestational period, were also distributed to pregnant women. However, as there is no systematic survey of data on micronutrient deficiencies in indigenous children and pregnant women, and the lack of micronutrients is only noted when health is seriously affected, the problem persists and the actions are palliative (UNICEF, 2006).

In a study carried out by Surui, Mariano and Rios (2014), nineteen children under the age of five in the villages that make up the Surui indigenous people, belonging to the Cacoal/RO Base Pole, were found to be malnourished in 2013. It should be noted that the authors did not specify the total number of children living in the villages, which makes it impossible to calculate a percentage of malnutrition in them.

The nutritionist responsible for monitoring the nutritional development of the children in this indigenous community points out issues related to the indigenous culture itself when she points out that the parents don't sit down with the children to eat and that they are fed after the parents, If food is offered and the child refuses, there is no insistence, which significantly worsens the state of malnutrition, which is already precarious due to the quality of the food (SURUI, MARIANO, RIOS, 2014).

As a measure to reduce malnutrition rates in these villages, the Ministry of Health then implemented, together with the DSEI and the Ministry of Social Development and Fight against Hunger, the PSFI strategy - Indigenous Family Health Program, which includes a nutritionist in its team, whose work focuses on prioritizing actions to prevent, promote and recover health in a comprehensive and continuous manner (SURUI, MARIANO, RIOS, 2014).

The distribution of food baskets was another strategy used, but this distribution is not punctual, which does not make the action effective, in addition to the lack of resources and staff turnover at the DSEI, which makes it impossible to continue the work. The nutritionist also reveals that the main actions were lectures given to the indigenous people, which, in her view, did not generate positive results, including the waste of food that came in the food baskets due to the indigenous people's lack of knowledge of how to use it. In view of this context, we started to provide guidance on how to make better use of the food produced in the villages, in different ways, such as preparing cakes, pies, polenta, etc. This action minimized the situation, but it wasn't enough. When children became ill due to food risks, they were sent to the Indigenous Health Houses (CASAI), where they remained until they recovered and stabilized, and were then sent back to their villages of origin. However, with the lack of care, the situation ended up repeating itself and the children systematically returned to the CASAI, with the authors considering that the objective was not fully achieved, as the problem was not solved but rather alleviated (SURUI, MARIANO, RIOS, 2014).

In the study by Kühl, Corso, Leite and Bastos (2009), it was found that the Kaingàng people, who live in the Mangueirinha Indigenous Territory, in the southwest of Paranà, also face serious problems in terms of health care, which invariably reflects on the nutritional status of indigenous children under the age of five, with malnutrition being one of the most common health problems and a cause of death.

In the survey, 141 children were assessed, out of a total of 147 living in the five villages that make up the Kaingàng people. It was observed that 95% of the children evaluated had some kind of parasite, mainly *Ascaris lumbricoides,* followed by *Entamoeba coli.* The authors refer to this serious situation.

[...] the precarious environmental and sanitary conditions to which the Kaingàng are generally exposed, such as the lack of water treatment, the use of reused material to build houses, the high family density, the lack of electricity, the absence of basic sanitation, the contamination of the soil by waste deposited in the open and the lack of garbage collection (KÜHL; CORSO; LEITE; BASTOS, 2009).

After anthropometric evaluation, the authors found that most of the children were already underweight at birth, which corroborates the research by Surui, Mariano and Rios (2014), revealing the lack of care since pregnancy and that the situation is only aggravated by poor dietary conditions and sanitary care, causing a high rate of malnutrition and parasitic diseases, causing comorbidities that can lead to death.

The research by Martins and Menezes (1994) was carried out in two Amazonian villages, Maroxewara and Paranatinga, with a total of eighty children and, of these, 33.8% had moderate and severe forms of malnutrition, with growth retardation.

The authors observed that the village that has had the longest contact with non-Indians has seen a significant change in its source of food and in the way it produces it. Before this contact, hunting, fishing and the planting of staple foods such as corn, manioc and other tubers, gave way to more marketable crops such as bananas, açai and Brazil nuts, for example, and the making of handicrafts for sale, since the village was close to the Transamazon highway, further impoverishing the type of food they ate and using the money raised from the sale of products to satisfy the needs created by the process of acculturation, such as clothes, cigarettes, industrialized foods and others (MARTINS; MENEZES, 1994).

This change in lifestyle and diet meant that malnutrition rates were even higher, prompting measures to be taken in primary care and other areas such as education and stimulating production, with the aim of reversing the situation. Malnutrition was reduced by 50%, but the authors point out that, as it is a social factor and not just a health issue, many actions still need to be taken to effectively put an end to malnutrition in the villages studied.

In his study, Santos (1993) emphasized the scarcity of studies, either by independent researchers or government entities, to delineate the physical growth patterns and nutritional status of indigenous populations.

This author, through his research, found that the short stature of indigenous children comes from the chronic malnutrition that affects most of them, caused by nutritional deficiencies and poor health conditions in the villages. He also emphasized that the reduction in dietary diversity caused by the abandonment of traditional subsistence practices and the occasional deficiencies in primary health care programs cause, in addition to malnutrition, a high prevalence of infectious and parasitic diseases, as previously mentioned in other studies (SANTOS, 1993).

Santos also stresses the importance of carrying out studies on the subject and promoting actions to monitor the child from pregnancy onwards, with special attention to the nutritional status of the pregnant woman and subsequent monitoring of the child in order to minimize the serious malnutrition that occurs in indigenous populations.

CONCLUSION

Malnutrition in indigenous children is still a significant reality in Brazil.

Through the readings carried out, it was found that the problem has always existed, but has worsened since the indigenous people came into contact with non-indigenous people, due to the process of acculturation, which removed important nutrients from their diet and introduced unhealthy habits, such as alcoholism, smoking, excessive consumption of industrialized products, since life in the villages no longer revolves around getting the best food for their subsistence, but on producing for sale, be it food or handicrafts, which means that the nutritional deficiencies of these populations are increasing more and more.

It was interesting to note that studies from the 1980s to the most recent ones report the same situations, both nutritional and social, and that the governmental actions taken to combat this scenario (malnutrition, better sanitary conditions, primary health care, etc.) are sparse and ineffective, either due to a lack of resources or a deficiency in the training of professionals trained to work specifically with indigenous populations.

Surui, Mariano and Rios (2014) point to the fact that there is a high turnover of professionals working in the villages, which does not allow for the creation of bonds and trust between the indigenous people and the professionals and vice versa, making it difficult to develop more effective work with better results.

It was also observed that there is no solid data on anthropometry in indigenous populations, which makes it difficult to establish their nutritional profile. Perhaps this fact can be attributed to the diversity of indigenous lands in Brazil, which would require many years of research and studies to map these populations in their entirety.

The fact is that malnutrition is a problem that, despite advances in the area of primary health care within indigenous reservations, there is still a lot of resistance from individuals and many deficiencies in the programs developed, so that the situation does not change significantly, with more forceful action only being taken when the indices go from serious to alarming, as in the case mentioned above in the states of Mato Grosso and Mato Grosso do Sul.

Establishing a nutritional profile of Brazilian indigenous children under the age of five is a task that has yet to be done, but which would be essential if we were to organize health actions to improve the current situation.

REFERENCES

ALTINI, Emilia; RODRIGUES, Gilderlan; PADILHA, Lindomar; MORAES, Paulo Daniel; LIEBGOTT, Roberto Antônio. **A Politica de Atençâo à Saùde Indigena no Brasil:** breve recuperação histórica sobre a política de assistência à saúde nas comunidades indigenas. Indigenous Missionary Council: São Paulo, 2013. Available at: http://6ccr.pgr.mpf.mp.br/institucional/grupos-de- trabalho/saude/cartilha-sobre-saude-indigena-cimi Accessed on 09/04/2016.

BRAZIL. Ministry of Health. National Health Foundation. **National**

atençâo à saùde dos povos indigenas. 2 ed. Brasilia: MS/FUNASA, 2002.

CHAGAS, Deysianne das; SILVA, Antonio Augusto Moura da; BATISTA, Rosangela Fernandes Lucena; SIMOES, Vanda Maria Ferreira; LAMY, Zeni Carvalho; COIMBRA, Liberata Campos; ALVES, Maria Teresa Seabra Soares de Britto e. Prevalence and factors associated with malnutrition and overweight in children under five in the six largest municipalities of Maranhao. **Rev Bras Epidemiol** 2013; 16(1): 146-56. Available at:

http://www.scielosp.org/pdf/rbepid/v16n1/1415-790X-rbepid-16-01 - 0146.pdf Accessed on 02/06/2016.

FERNANDES, Benedito Scaranci. A new approach to the serious problem of child malnutrition. **Estud. Av.** vol.17 no.48 Sâo Paulo May/Aug. 2003. Available at :

http://www.scielo.br/scielo.php?script=sci arttext&pid=S0103-

40142003000200007 Accessed on 03/06/2016.

GIL, Antonio Carlos. **Methods and techniques of social research**. 6. ed. - Sâo Paulo: Atlas, 2008.

JONSSON, Urban. The causes of hunger. In: **Hunger and malnutrition**: social determinants. Sâo Paulo: Cortez, 1986.

LAKATOS, Eva Maria; MARCONI, Marina de Andrade. **Metodologia cientifica**. 4- ed. Sâo Paulo: Atlas, 2006.

MARTINS, Sandro J.; MENEZES, Raiumundo. Evoluçao do estado nutricional de menores de 5 anos em aldeias indigenas da Tribo Parakana, na Amazônia Oriental Brasileira (1989-1991). **Rev. Saùde Pùblica** vol.28 no.1 Sao Paulo Feb. 1994. Available at: http://www.scielo.br/scielo.php?script=sci arttext&pid=S0034-89101994000100001 Accessed on 03/06/2016.

MOURA, Alice Bezerra de Mello. **The national health care policy for indigenous peoples**. 2012. Available at:

http://www.ufpe.br/remdipe/index.php?option=com content&view=article&id=395&Itemid=251 Accessed on 12/04/2016.

SANTOS, Ricardo V. Physical growth and nutritional status of Brazilian indigenous populations. **Cad. Saùde Pùblica** vol.9 suppl.1 Rio de Janeiro 1993. Available at: http://www.scielo.br/scielo.php?script=sci arttext&pid=S0102- 311X1993000500006 Accessed on 13/06/2016.

SURUI, Karen Walenepanhie G.; MARIANO, Vanessa Thomasi; RIOS, Mirivan Carneiro. **Child malnutrition among indigenous peoples of the Surui ethnic group in the municipality of Cacoal/RO**. 2014. Available at: http://www.unifia.edu.br/revista eletronica/revistas/saude foco/artig os/ano2014/desnutricao infantil.pdf Accessed on 12/05/2016.

UNICEF. **Malnutrition**: a threat to health. 2006. Available at: http://www.unicef.org/brazil/pt/Pags 040 051 Malnutrition.pdf Accessed on 13/05/2016.

4. DISEASES ACQUIRED BY THE INDIGENOUS POPULATION THROUGH CONTACT WITH THE NON-INDIGENOUS POPULATION

Dione Scarabelot Gomes, Clóvis Luciano Giacomet

INTRODUCTION

The diseases acquired by indigenous populations when they come into contact with non-indigenous populations, considering that the indigenous, in a cultural way, have their own ways of taking care of their illnesses, curing their illnesses and even worsening their illnesses. The question was: what dangers do the diseases of the "white population" pose to indigenous communities? This question has been answered throughout the development of this material. The theme raised stems from reflections on the subject that establish that the health of indigenous peoples, since the colonization of Brazil and the contact of the indigenous with the "white population", has suffered important impacts, from its epidemiological profile to the model of indigenous health care. Infectious and contagious diseases occupy a very important place in the life history of indigenous people and are the main causes of death and illness in their populations. Before the country was colonized, the diseases known to the indigenous communities that inhabited Brazil were venomous animal bites, diarrhea, poisoning from eating poisonous plants, wounds caused by hunting and routine activities. These were diseases that the indigenous people knew how to treat with their own natural medicine.

Today it is known that many medicinal plants and many remedies from them have been learned, scientifically proven and today patented and marketed by the pharmaceutical industries, many at very high costs.

When they came into contact with the non-Indians, they came across diseases that were unknown to them until then and which decimated them and continue to kill indigenous people to this day: measles, flu, malaria, variola, chickenpox, hepatitis and Sexually Transmitted Diseases (gonorrhea, syphilis, warts).

Sex diseases appeared in indigenous communities through contact with the colonizers, as well as influenza, a simple disease caused by a virus that does not cause major health complications for the non-indigenous population, but which, when it came into contact with indigenous populations, decimated them due to the lack of immunity of these populations, who were previously unaware of this disease.

In 1960, millions of indigenous Brazilians, when they came into contact with rubber tappers in the Amazon, died from an outbreak of influenza, which at the time was considered an epidemic among the indigenous population.

INDIGENOUS HEALTH CARE AND ITS IMPACTS

The history of the Brazilian Indians begins with the accounts given by Pero Vaz de Caminha on the arrival of Pedro Alvares Cabral's expedition to Brazil, which, according to history, lost its way to the Indies, on the Asian continent, in search of gold, precious stones and spices.

There began the decimation of a people who, before the arrival of the non-Indians, lived in an organized and structured society, divided into tribes according to the region they inhabited.

Each tribe had its own way of life, where the men were generally responsible for hunting, fishing and making tools for these purposes, and the women and children for gathering fruit and seeds, making tools and maintaining the huts. There was also a clear hierarchy to be respected, in the form of chiefs, shamans and elders who were extremely respected. Their customs and beliefs were based on elements of nature and, as such, they worshipped these elements as gods, namely the sun, rain, thunder, etc.

They also fought for territory and defended their tribe from others and from animals that might pose a threat. Their illnesses were cured by the shaman, the tribe's healer, using herbs and roots. Until then, not many diseases affecting non-Indians from civilized continents were known.

According to Fausto (1996):

With contact with non-Indians, in addition to the process of acculturation, also came diseases such as measles, variola and influenza, against which the Indians had no resistance, decimating thousands of them. Two epidemic waves stood out for their violence between 1562 and 1563, killing more than 60,000 Indians, it seems, not counting the victims of the serfdom. The death of the indigenous population, which was partly dedicated to planting food crops, resulted in a terrible famine in the Northeast and a loss of arms.

None of the initiatives related to the care of indigenous populations took into account the specificity of this population, ignoring their values, representations and practices related to health and illness, demonstrating a lack of respect for the context of the indigenous individual's relationship with society and the environment in which they lived.

According to Langdon (2005):

In 1967, the Service for the Protection of Indians and National Workers was abolished and FUNAI (the National Indian Foundation) was created, along with the Volante Health Teams, which provided sporadic care to the indigenous communities in their area of coverage, providing medical assistance, administering vaccines and supervising the work of the local health personnel, who were limited to nursing assistants and attendants.

However, this service fell into decline after the financial crisis that hit Brazil in the 1970s, causing resources for care to become scarce, making the services provided even more precarious, in addition to the extinction of the Volante Health Teams, which ended up dissolving due to a lack of professionals who ended up settling in urban centers and in administrative activities, returning to a model of emergency and palliative care, provided by people with little qualification.

Since then, discussions have taken place in order to structure a system capable of offering more effective and punctual health care to the indigenous population, as was the case with the First National Conference for the Protection of Indigenous Health and the Second National Conference on Health for Indigenous Peoples, which took place in 1986 and 1993 respectively, on the recommendation of the Eighth and Ninth National Health Conferences. These two Conferences proposed the structuring of a differentiated care model, based on the strategy of Special Indigenous Health Districts, as a way of guaranteeing indigenous peoples the right to universal and comprehensive access to health, meeting the needs perceived by the communities and involving the indigenous population in all stages of the planning, implementation and evaluation of actions. In 1991, as part of the actions guided by the above-mentioned Conferences, through a decree, the government transferred responsibility for coordinating health actions aimed at indigenous populations to the Ministry of Health, establishing the Special Indigenous Health Districts as the basis for organizing health services. The Ministry of Health then created the Coordination of Indigenous Health (COSAI), which was responsible for implementing a new model of indigenous health care (BRASIL, 2002).

Even with important actions, Brazil has not managed to establish important actions to promote and combat indigenous diseases.

Indigenous diseases which, in contact with non-Indian populations, have no immunity or forms of control.

INDIGENOUS DISEASES ACQUIRED THROUGH CONTACT WITH NON-INDIANS

The many diseases that have decimated indigenous populations acquired through contact with non-indigenous populations have always caused major health problems for the entire community affected by these diseases.

According to Brasil (2002):

Among the indigenous populations, the most frequent morbidities are acute respiratory and gastrointestinal infections, malaria, tuberculosis, sexually transmitted diseases, malnutrition and vaccine-preventable diseases, showing a health situation characterized by the high occurrence of diseases that could be significantly reduced with the establishment of systematic and continuous basic health care actions within the indigenous areas. In addition to these problems, in regions where the indigenous population maintains a closer relationship with the local population (which is becoming more and more common), we can see the emergence of health problems related to changes in the way of life, especially in diet, usually causing hypertension, diabetes, cancer, alcoholism and depression, drawing attention to the frightening rise in the number of suicides in these populations.

Contact with other populations of non-Indian origin leads to a change in lifestyle habits and also in diet. *The* consumption of canned products with high doses of lipids, glycerides and glucose also affects the health of indigenous populations.

According to Botelho (2008):

Currently, the incidence of diabetes mellitus in the white population is two per thousand inhabitants per year. Among Indians, this proportion is absurdly higher, reaching more than 30 cases per thousand inhabitants per year. The Brazilian, Mexican and Andean populations, with a mixture of whites and Indians, are also affected and are more prone to obesity and diabetes.

The change in lifestyle and eating habits has led to the emergence of diseases in the indigenous population that a few years ago were only common in non-Indian urban populations, such as diabetes and obesity.

CHANGES IN INDIGENOUS HABITS

Carbohydrates are high-calorie foods with a high glycemic index that increase the risk of heart disease and diabetes. In indigenous populations, the increase in cases of diabetes and heart disease is related to excessive consumption of carbohydrates.

As Botelho (2008) explains:

Among the factors that have led to the current rates of obesity and diabetes among indigenous Brazilians are genetic predisposition and the loss of food culture in the villages, as well as sedentary lifestyles. As a result of contact with urban areas and access to commercialized items, the indigenous people gradually abandoned their routine of hunting and gathering and cultivating small plots of food such as manioc, carà, pumpkin, sweet potato, beans and corn, among others.

Obesity in indigenous groups is a factor that triggers many diseases, and the biggest problem is that it is often not seen as a disease, but only as an aesthetic problem. Obesity in indigenous peoples manifests itself when these groups begin to consume industrialized products, taking into account their genetic predisposition to fat accumulation.

For Vergara (1998):

According to João Botelho - a pioneer in describing the incidence of diabetes mellitus among Brazilian Indians, during nearly 30 years of studying indigenous health - "crystallized sugar and sucrose, constant in the white man's diet, are highly toxic to Indians. "

The food consumed by non-indigenous groups not only causes illness but also affects indigenous culture, one of the most important elements of which is the healing of illnesses through plants and medicinal remedies.

This indigenous knowledge about medicinal plants and cures is becoming extinct over the generations, which reflects a great loss of knowledge and culture not only for the indigenous people, but for all the peoples who make use of this knowledge in some way. **THE PROCESS OF INDIGENOUS ACCULTURATION AND DISEASES**

The history of the Brazilian Indians begins with the accounts of Pero Vaz de Caminha when Pedro Alvares Cabral's expedition arrived in Brazil. According to history, he got lost on the way to the Indies, on the Asian continent, in search of gold, precious stones and spices.

There began the decimation of a people who, before the arrival of the non-Indians, lived in an organized and structured society, in their own way, divided into tribes according to the region in which they lived.

Each tribe had its own way of life, where the men were generally responsible for hunting, fishing and making tools for these purposes, and the women and children for gathering fruit and seeds, making tools and maintaining the huts.

There was also a clear hierarchy to be respected, in the form of chiefs, shamans and elders who were extremely respected. Their customs and beliefs were based on elements of nature and, as such, they worshipped these elements as gods, namely the sun, rain, thunder, etc.

They also fought for territory and defended their tribe from others and from animals that might pose a threat. Their illnesses were cured by the shaman, the tribe's healer, using herbs and roots. Until then, not many diseases affecting non-Indians from civilized continents were known.

Realizing that the indigenous people were docile and easily manipulated, they began to be used as labour and treated inhumanely, because, for the Portuguese, they didn't have souls and therefore didn't deserve any humane treatment. The brandy given to the "uncivilized and uncultured" people was to anesthetize them so that they would be able to carry out the hard day's work. Those who didn't know the value of gold, precious metals or the wood that would produce a dye with a high commercial value would be given newly produced strong brandy so that drunkards could be treated like worthless, uncultured animals. In this way, they would be "domesticated and civilized" more easily and would repay the "chiefs and owners of the new land" for their attempts to make them "human". Thus, along with the colonizers came slavery, the seizure of land and precious metals, as well as new customs and new diseases.

Fever, tetanus, hemeralopia, tenesmus, opilation, spasms, variola, measles, influenza, yellow fever, malaria, typhus, tuberculosis, are some of the many diseases that affected and still affect the indigenous population after the colonization process.

The fever probably alluded to various illnesses, with the patient suffering from headaches and high body temperatures.

Snake bites and venomous animals posed great risks to life and the Indians fell victim to tetanus, pain, infections and mutilations.

Hemeralopia, an eye disease that caused blurred vision and, in more serious cases, blindness.

Tenesmus manifests as a painful sensation in the bladder or anal region, with a continuous but almost useless urge to urinate or defecate.

Spasms are characterized by the loss of the ability to breathe and swallow, believed to be a "convulsion of the diaphragm and esophagus", and by the emission of "a horrible murmur, in the manner of epileptics.

Variola came to the American continent from Europe with Columbus. It is considered one of the main factors responsible for the distribution of the native populations of America.

Measles made its appearance in Brazil from the beginning of settlement and colonization. Brought by the black African and European populations, it is very similar to chickenpox and its most obvious characteristic is the rash on the skin.

It is very difficult to gather exact historical data on influenza, as its symptoms are similar to those of other diseases, such as diphtheria, typhoid fever, dengue fever or typhus.

Yellow fever is a disease characteristic of wild areas, forests and savannahs. Found in Central and South America as well as Africa, its symptoms include high fever, foul-smelling diarrhea, convulsions and delirium, internal bleeding and disseminated intravascular coagulation, with damage and infarction in various organs. The hemorrhages manifest as bleeding from the nose and gums and ecchymoses (blue or green spots of clotted blood on the skin). Hepatitis also occurs and sometimes fatal shock due to heavy bleeding into internal body cavities. These diseases have claimed many Brazilian victims.

Malaria is an acute or chronic infectious disease.

Typhus, transmitted by lice or fleas and characterized by fevers and a drop in blood pressure, was often confused with malaria, due to the difficulty at the time in diagnosing and distinguishing diseases followed by fevers. In many regions of the country, these diseases still claim many victims in indigenous communities.

CONCLUSION

The problem of Brazilian indigenous people with regard to the promotion and maintenance of health has been flawed since the colonization of Brazil, since the actions developed are sporadic and disorganized in the sense of implementing a public policy that really meets the needs of this population, taking into account all the specificities of the various ethnic groups that make up the various indigenous societies spread throughout the national territory.

It was also found that the causes of many diseases were related to contact with the white population. Initially. In addition, associated pathologies such as hypertension, malaria, depression and others, which were previously unknown to the indigenous people, are now common and have become a serious public health problem that deserves a closer look from health agencies, especially those responsible for indigenous societies.

From what has been raised, it is possible to conclude that the change in the lifestyle of Brazil's indigenous populations is a serious public health problem and that more specific actions need to be considered in order to concretely minimize this problem and offer decent living conditions for these populations that have been marginalized since the colonization of Brazil.

REFERENCES

BOTELHO, J.A. **Saùde indigena**. Rio de Janeiro: Editores Associados, 2008.

BRAZIL. **National Survey on Alcohol Consumption Patterns in the Brazilian Population**. National Anti-Drugs Secretariat, 2007. Available at:

http://bvsms.saude.gov.br/bvs/publicacoes/relatorio_alcohol_consumption patterns.pdf Accessed on 01/02/2015

. **Law n. 6001, of December 19, 1973**. Provides for the Statute of the Indian. Brazil. 2009. Available at: http://www.funai.gov.br/eventos/30anos.htm Accessed on 29/02/2015.

. National Secretariat for Drug Policy. Brazilian report

FAUSTO, B. História **do Brasil covers a period of more than five hundred years, from the roots of Portuguese colonization to the present day**. EDUSP. 1996. Available at:

http://www.caccto.com.br/material/d00044/Material 6 EMED 2A 195641.pdf Accessed on 05/03/2015.

GIL, A. C. **Métodos e técnicas da pesquisa social.** *Sao* Paulo: 1987.

LANGDON, E. J. M. Alcohol abuse among indigenous peoples in Brazil: a comparative evaluation. **Tellus Magazine**. Campo Grande, ano 5 n.8/9 p.103-124 abr./out. 2005. Available at: http://neppi.ucdb.br/pub/tellus/tellus8_9/TL8e9 Esther Jean Langd on.pdf Accessed on 26/01/2015

VERGARA S. C. **Projetos e relatórios de pesquisa em administraçâo.** Sao Paulo: Atlas, 1998.

5. INDIGENOUS ORAL HEALTH CARE IN BRAZIL

Eduardo Ferraz Ribeiro do Valle Neto, Clóvis Luciano Giacomet

INTRODUCTION

According to Medeiros and Abreu (2006), the First National Health Conference, held in 1986, already established that oral health is an integral and inseparable part of the general health of the human organism. Many diseases of the body show signs in the mouth, which can be significant indications of general health problems.

It is therefore very important that oral health is an integral part of the population's health care programs, with the aim of preventing oral problems that end up affecting health in general.

As far as public policies are concerned, prior to 2004, oral health actions were offered in parallel to the process of organizing other services, therefore, in a random manner, without effectiveness and with low resolving power, so that they were unable to solve or minimize the main oral health problems of the population.

In 2004, the federal government launched, through the Ministry of Health, the "National Oral Health Policy - Smiling Brazil", through which oral health began to be offered in an integral way, together with Primary Health Care and the creation of a network of oral health care services in the Unified Health System - SUS, with the aim of rescuing the citizenship of the Brazilian population.

In 2011, the Ministry of Health's General Coordination of Oral Health concluded the fourth nationwide epidemiological survey in the area of oral health, with the aim of understanding the reality and planning new actions to improve the quality of the population's oral health.

Indigenous communities were also included in the program, with the Indigenous Smiling Program, which aims to expand access to dental care in Brazil's indigenous villages, structuring and qualifying oral health services in the Special Indigenous Health Districts (DSEIs).

Given that the author of this paper works as a dental professional in an indigenous village, there was an interest in researching the subject, learning about existing public policies, with the aim of demonstrating their importance as a form of basic care for indigenous populations.

In order to achieve this goal, bibliographic research was used, searching for references on research sites such as *Scielo* and BVS - Biblioteca Virtual em Saùde (Virtual Health Library), as well as official *sites* such as the Ministry of Health, FUNASA and FUNAI, to collect data, using the following descriptors: oral health, oral health care, indigenous oral health, public policies on oral health.

PUBLIC POLICIES RELATING TO INDIGENOUS PEOPLE IN BRAZIL

According to FUNASA (2002), since the beginning of Portuguese colonization, the indigenous people were cared for by the missionaries in an integrated way with government policies. At the beginning of the 20th century, with territorial and economic expansion, which brought with it the construction of railroad and telegraph lines, there were numerous massacres of indigenous peoples and a huge rise in mortality rates from communicable diseases, This led to the creation, in 1910, of the Service for the Protection of Indians and National Workers, which was attached to the Ministry of Agriculture and whose aim was to protect Indians and progressively integrate their lands into the national production system.

However, the indigenous people were still seen as individuals in evolution, considered to be at an infantile stage of humanity and the assistance provided was sporadic and disorganized, limited to emergency or "pacifist" actions. This situation lasted until the 1950s, with no public policies aimed at systematic care, which resulted in many deaths from infectious and contagious diseases that affected the indigenous populations, until the creation of the Air Sanitary Units Service, which aimed to bring health actions to populations in areas that were difficult to access, essentially focused on vaccination, dental care, tuberculosis control and other communicable diseases (BRASIL, 2002).

In 1967, the Service for the Protection of Indians and National Workers was abolished and FUNAI and the Volante Health Teams were created, which provided sporadic assistance to the indigenous communities in their area of coverage, providing medical care, administering vaccines and supervising the work of the health personnel in these locations, who were limited to nursing assistants and attendants. However, this service fell into decline after the financial crisis that hit Brazil in the 1970s, causing resources for care to become scarce, further compromising the services provided, in addition to the extinction of the Volante Health Teams, which ended up dissolving due to a lack of professionals who ended up settling in urban centers and in administrative activities, returning to a model of emergency and palliative care, provided by people with little qualification.

It is noteworthy that none of the initiatives related to the care of indigenous populations took into account the specificity of this population, ignoring their values, their representations and practices related to health and illness, demonstrating disrespect for the context of the indigenous individual's relations with society and the environment in which they lived.

The situation described only changed with the 1988 Constitution, which "stipulated the recognition and respect of the socio-cultural organizations of indigenous peoples, assuring them full civil capacity - making the institution of guardianship obsolete - and established the exclusive competence of the Union to legislate and deal with indigenous issues" (BRASIL, 2002). The Constitution also defined the general principles of the Unified Health System (SUS), later regulated by Law 8.080/90, and established that the sole direction and responsibility for the federal management of the system lies with the Ministry of Health.

From then on, discussions took place in order to structure a system capable of offering more effective and timely health care to the indigenous population, as was the case with the First National Conference on the Protection of Indigenous Health and the Second National Conference on Health for Indigenous Peoples, which took place in 1986 and 1993 respectively, on the recommendation of the Eighth and Ninth National Health Conferences.

These two Conferences proposed the structuring of a differentiated model of care, based on the strategy of Special Indigenous Health Districts, as a way of guaranteeing indigenous peoples the right to universal and comprehensive access to health, meeting the needs perceived by the communities and involving the indigenous population in all stages of the process of planning, executing and evaluating actions (BRASIL, 2002).

In 1991, as part of the actions guided by the above-mentioned Conferences, by means of a decree, the government transferred to the Ministry of Health the responsibility for coordinating health actions aimed at indigenous populations, establishing the Special Indigenous Health Districts as the basis for organizing health services. The Ministry of Health then created the Coordination of Indigenous Health (COSAI), which was responsible for implementing a new model of indigenous health care (BRASIL, 2002).

In the same year, Resolution 11, of October 13, 1991, of the National Health Council (CNS), created the Inter-Sectoral Commission on

Indigenous Health (CISI), whose main task was to advise the CNS on the development of principles and guidelines for government policies in the field of indigenous health.

However, in 1994, also by presidential decree, the coordination of health actions was returned to FUNAI, delegating responsibility for the recovery of the health of sick indigenous people and prevention to the Ministry of Health, which would be responsible for immunization, sanitation, human resources training and endemic disease control.

This defragmentation of the indigenous health care model meant that responsibility was divided between FUNASA and FUNAI, causing a "breakdown" in the care provided to the populations, since the actions were disconnected and individual.

In 1997, the Inter-Sectoral Commission on Indigenous Health of the National Health Council (CISI/CNS) requested the intervention of the Federal Public Prosecutor's Office (6- CCR/MPF) because of the federal government's failure to implement an adequate policy for indigenous health care. The public hearing held in November 1997 concluded that the responsibility established in the Federal Constitution for indigenous health care lay with the Ministry of Health at the federal level, and that "the refusal of institutions linked to the SUS to provide this assistance constituted an illegal act that could be confronted through the competent channels" (ALTINI, et.al., 2013).

As a result of the increased pressure, in 1999 the federal government issued Decree No. 3.156 and promoted the approval of the "Arouca Law" (Law No. 9.836, of September 23, 1999) in the National Congress. This law was written by Congressman Sérgio Arouca, one of the leaders of the Health Reform, regulating the guidelines approved at the Second National Conference on Indigenous Health, and had been shelved in Congress since 1994. Indigenous health policy became the exclusive responsibility of the Ministry of Health: "The Ministry of Health will establish the policies and guidelines for the promotion, prevention and recovery of indigenous health, whose actions will be carried out by FUNASA". The Arouca Law ordered the federal government to set up the Indigenous Health Care Subsystem (SASI-SUS), based on the Special Indigenous Health Districts (DSEIs). The 34 DSEIs were then created through Ordinance 852/1999 (ALTINI, et.al, 2013).

In view of the serious health problems faced by indigenous peoples, in 1999 the federal government sanctioned Law No. 9.836, adding provisions to Law No. 8.080, of 1990, laying down the conditions for the promotion, protection and recovery of health, the organization and operation of the corresponding services in relation to indigenous populations, establishing, at that time, the Indigenous Health Care Subsystem, which is linked to the Department of Indigenous Health Care, which, according to Moura (2012), has:

[...] the mission of planning, coordinating and supervising comprehensive health care activities for indigenous peoples; guiding and supporting the implementation of health care programs for the indigenous population, according to SUS guidelines; planning, coordinating and supervising health education activities in the Special Indigenous Health Districts; coordinating the development of norms and guidelines for the operationalization of health care actions in the Special Indigenous Health Districts; providing technical advice to the teams of the Special Indigenous Health Districts in the development of health care actions; support the preparation of District Indigenous Health Plans and coordinate building and environmental sanitation actions within the Special Indigenous Health Districts.

According to MS Ordinance No. 2607, of December 10, 2004, the Special Indigenous Health Districts are a model for organizing services, which include a set of technical activities, aimed at rationalized and qualified health care measures, promoting the reorganization of the health network and health practices and developing administrative-managerial activities necessary for the provision of care, with social control.

Also in 2009, the 34 Special Indigenous Health Districts (DSEIs) were given administrative autonomy. The DSEIs became decentralized management units, responsible for health care and basic sanitation in each region. The autonomy of the districts reduces bureaucracy in indigenous health care, which is now integrated and articulated with the entire Unified Health System (SUS) (BRASIL, 2002).

In 2004, FUNASA, through ordinances 69 and 70, established new guidelines for indigenous health, with the aim of recovering direct execution and reducing the role of the contracted organizations, limiting them to hiring staff, providing care in the villages with supplies, moving indigenous people from the villages, and buying fuel for these trips. In 2006, the Fòrum de Presidentes dos Conselhos Distritais de Saùde Indigena (Forum of Presidents of District Indigenous Health Councils) was set up to act in an advisory and propositional capacity, in line with the other decision-making bodies of the SUS (BRASIL, 2002).

In the process of holding the fourth National Conference on Indigenous Health in 2006, several district conferences presented the proposal to create a Special Secretariat for Indigenous Health (SESAI), due to the worsening of the recurring problems of mismanagement, authoritarianism, political use and corruption in FUNASA's regional coordinations and central bodies. This proposal was taken to the plenary of the national stage of the conference, and ended up being defeated by a small margin of votes, prompting many of the indigenous delegations to denounce the manipulation of the conference proceedings (ALTINI, et.al, 2013).

On October 17, 2007, FUNASA issued the controversial Ordinance No. 2.656, which regulated the Incentives for Basic and Specialized Care for Indigenous Peoples, revoking Ordinance No. 1.633/GM of September 14, 1999. This decree generated huge protests from indigenous peoples, dissatisfied with the policy that FUNASA was managing, who demanded the creation of a policy model compatible with the Arouca Law and the guidelines of the Second National Conference on Indigenous Health. As well as strengthening FUNASA, the ordinance opened up concrete prospects for the municipalization of indigenous health, exactly the opposite of what the indigenous peoples wanted.

It was only in August 2008, after constant demonstrations by the indigenous movement against FUNASA, and countless accusations of corruption and neglect in the execution of actions and services in indigenous areas, which had been generating overwhelming infant mortality and the spread of diseases, that the Minister of Health decided to listen to the complaints and proposals of the indigenous peoples.

During this same period, the Federal Court of Auditors (TCU) carried out an audit of FUNASA, focusing on issues relating to the management of indigenous health policy. At the same time, the Labor Court ruled that the federal government was responsible and therefore the manager of the health policy, and that outsourcing was an illegal practice.

At the end of 2008, Bill No. 3.958 was presented with a view to amending Law No. 10.683/2003, which deals with the organization of the Presidency of the Republic and the Ministries, and creating the Secretariat for Primary Care and Health Promotion, which would house indigenous health. In the bill's explanatory statement, the Minister of Health proposed transferring Funasa's powers and responsibilities to this secretariat. Also as a result of pressure from indigenous peoples, a

Working Group was set up with the participation of indigenous leaders (ordinances 3.034/2008 and 3.035/2008 - GAB/MS), whose aim was to discuss and present proposals, actions and measures to be implemented within the Ministry of Health, with regard to the management of health services offered to indigenous peoples.

After two years of waiting, the government issued Provisional Measure No. 483, which was approved by Congress and transformed into Law No. 12.314/2010. On October 19, 2010, Decree No. 7.336/2010 was issued, making official the creation of the Special Secretariat for Indigenous Health (SESAI). This transitional period for the implementation of the new management of indigenous health was characterized by shared management between SESAI and Funasa, and although the government had set a deadline of three months for detailing its structure and other measures to make it operational, the situation dragged on for more than three years while health care in the communities went through critical moments.

At the end of 2012, the Articulation of Indigenous Peoples of Brazil (APIB) published a letter to the Minister of Health expressing the growing outcry of indigenous leaders, communities and organizations from all over Brazil, and their indignation at the worrying state of chaos and calamity in which indigenous health care has become, in conditions similar to those at the time of the management of the National Health Foundation (Funasa). The document called for an effective intervention in SESAI so that it could actually fulfil its mission, in accordance with the expectations placed in it since its creation as a result of the struggle of Brazil's indigenous peoples and organizations.

Today, from an indigenous population estimated at 5 million at the time of the colonization of Brazil, there are only 370,000 Indians living in all Brazilian states, with the exception of Piaui and Rio Grande do Norte, divided into around 210 peoples, speaking 170 different languages, occupying around 12% of the Brazilian territory, a portion of whom live in urban areas, usually on the outskirts (BRASIL, 2002).

Also according to FUNASA (2002), many of these peoples are threatened with disappearance, and among some of them biological reproduction has been compromised, such is the reduction in population, as is the case in the state of Rondônia, where intense logging, mining and farming activities have caused extremely high mortality, with an estimated population of 6,284 people in 1999, remnants of 22 peoples, is one example of this. While some of these societies are undergoing a process of population recovery, like the Pakaas Novos, for example, who today number more than 2,000, others, like the Latundê, have suffered a process of reduction and currently number just 37 people.

Among the indigenous population, the most frequent morbidities are acute respiratory and gastrointestinal infections, malaria, tuberculosis, sexually transmitted diseases, malnutrition and vaccine-preventable diseases, showing a health situation characterized by the high occurrence of diseases that could be significantly reduced with the establishment of systematic and continuous primary health care actions within indigenous areas (BRASIL, 2002).

In addition to these problems, in regions where the indigenous population maintains a closer relationship with the local population (which is increasingly common), health problems related to changes in the way of life, especially in diet, are appearing, usually causing hypertension, diabetes, cancer, alcoholism and depression, drawing attention to the frightening rise in the number of suicides in these populations (BRASIL, 2002).

BASIC ORAL HEALTH CARE FOR INDIGENOUS POPULATIONS

Oral health is a determining factor for quality of life and personal development and, according to the World Health Organization, political, economic, social, cultural, environmental, behavioral and biological factors can improve or harm it (HIROOKA, 2010).

In relation to indigenous populations, studies on oral health are sparse and, due to the multiplicity of approaches, it is difficult to make a comparison between the research considering the methodological differences, age groups examined, dental care models, among others, showing that there is a gap to be filled in terms of scientific studies in the area (HIROOKA, 2010).

In the studies by Hirooka (2010), it was possible to identify the process of acculturation of indigenous people in the face of increasingly constant coexistence with non-indigenous culture, which leads to a significant change, especially in the eating habits of these peoples. The impact of this factor, combined with socio-economic and environmental changes, as well as the lack or deficiency of preventive programs, considerably increases the incidence of tooth decay and other oral health problems among indigenous peoples.

The author also mentions that a lower prevalence of oral health problems was observed among peoples who had less contact with non-indigenous societies, as they maintained more traditional characteristics (HIROOKA, 2010).

Another study, carried out by Souza and Ferreira (2012), showed that Brazil's indigenous populations comprise approximately 800,000 people, who belong to 220 peoples and speak 180 languages, whose health programs emphasize the organization of services, the provision of infrastructure and attempts at epidemiological surveys, which are the pillars of a Western medical model that aims to cure mainly the physical component of the disease.

These authors also highlight the scarcity of studies in the field of dentistry aimed at indigenous populations and, above all, the lack of the indigenous person's own view of the health-disease process and oral health problems.

In addition, they also cite the changes that have occurred as a result of living with non-indigenous people, especially with regard to food and the approach of the health professionals who serve these peoples, since there is a preoccupation with a curative approach rather than a preventive approach to general health problems and oral health specifically (SOUZA; FERREIRA, 2012).

Arantes (2005) also researched the oral health of indigenous peoples, more specifically the Xavantes of Mato Grosso, reporting that action in the area of oral health is neither systematized nor effective, which can be explained, according to him, by the high turnover of professionals who work in the programs developed, making it impossible to trace an epidemiological profile or the care provided.

INDIAN SMILING BRAZIL PROGRAM

The Brasil Sorridente Indigena Program is part of the National Oral Health Program launched by the federal government in 2003, which emerged as an alternative for improving health care for the Brazilian population, making it possible to carry out joint actions, since oral health demands are intrinsically linked to systemic diseases and providing oral health means providing general health.

According to the National Oral Health Policy, the main objective of this program is to reduce social exclusion and provide access to dental care for less privileged Brazilians, as a way of restoring citizenship (PNSB, BRASIL, 2004).

The National Oral Health Policy states that it is:

[...] it is essential to think about 'lines of care' (for children, adolescents, adults and the elderly), with the creation of flows that imply resolutive actions by the health teams, centered on welcoming, informing, assisting and referring (reference and counter-reference).

In this way, users can access and learn about each place that makes up the structure of the service through their experiences in it, making them feel part of it.

This line of care allows the process to be redirected and teamwork becomes the most important foundation, as it enables the team to get in tune with the universe of users and the emergence of bonds of trust and, consequently, a bond, which is indispensable for improving the quality of health services and the humanization of practices (PNSB, Brazil, 2004).

In the field of care, these guidelines point fundamentally to the expansion and qualification of primary care, enabling access to all age groups and the provision of more services, ensuring care at secondary and tertiary levels in order to seek comprehensive care (PNSB, Brazil, 2004).

In this way, the National Oral Health Policy, the Smiling Brazil Program, comprises a set of actions at the individual and collective levels that include health promotion, disease prevention, diagnosis, treatment and rehabilitation. This policy is developed through the exercise of democratic and participatory practices, in the form of teamwork, aimed at populations for whom responsibility for oral health care is assumed, taking into account the dynamics of the territory in which these populations live (BRASIL, 2004).

The Brasil Sorridente Indigena Program, an integral part of the National

Oral Health Policy coordinated by the Special Secretariat for Indigenous Health (SESAI) and the Secretariat for Health Care (SAS), aims to eliminate dental needs in indigenous villages throughout the country.

Its aim is to expand access to dental care in the villages, structuring and qualifying oral health services in the Special Indigenous Health Districts (DSEI), making it the first national policy designed specifically to deal with the oral health of these peoples.

The measures provided for in Brasil Sorridente Indigena are coordinated by the Ministry of Health and implemented by the DSEIs. The Health District is the central unit of the Indigenous Health Care Subsystem. It is responsible for technical and qualified primary health care activities. In Brazil, there are 34 units, which are not divided by state, but strategically based on the geographical occupation of indigenous communities. In addition to the DSEIs, the service structure includes health posts, Polos Bases and Casas de Saúde do Indio (CASAIS).

In this way, the Program has 26 dental surgeons, 11 oral health assistants (ASB) and 10 oral health technicians, as well as 74,000 oral hygiene kits, consisting of adult/child toothbrushes and fluoride toothpaste. More recently, it has also been able to count on 25 Mobile Dental Units, each of which has the capacity to carry out 350 consultations a month, demonstrating the high investments made in the Program.

According to FUNASA, the results of the program have been quite satisfactory, but it still needs to be expanded to serve a greater number of indigenous people, since these services are concentrated in just three centers.

CONCLUSION

From this research, it emerged that primary health care for indigenous people is still quite recent and that it took the struggle of many people for a health care policy to be created.

With regard to oral health, it was found that prior to 2003, i.e. before the Brasil Sorridente Indigena Program, the indigenous populations had little or no dental care and proof of this is the scant scientific production on the subject.

Since 2003, with the implementation of the National Oral Health Policy, care has been extended to the population in general and to specific populations, with investments in the area aimed at reducing the social exclusion to which these populations have been relegated since the arrival of the Portuguese colonizers in Brazil.

This is an important initiative to increase indigenous people's access to dental care in an effective and systematic way, so that they can preserve their health.

REFERENCES

ALTINI, E.; RODRIGUES, G.; PADILHA, L.; MORAES, P. DI; LIEBGOTT, R. A. **A Politica de Atençâo à Saùde Indigena no Brasil:** breve recuperação histórica sobre a política de assistência à saúde nas comunidades indigenas. Indigenous Missionary Council: São Paulo, 2013. Available at: http://6ccr.pgr.mpf.mp.br/institucional/grupos-de-trabalho/saude/cartilha-sobre-saude-indigena-cimi Accessed in 16/04/2016.

ARANTES, Rui. **Oral health of Brazil's indigenous peoples and the case of the Xavantes of Mato Grosso**. 2005. Available at: http://www.arca.fiocruz.br/bitstream/icict/4454/2/243.pdf Accessed on 20/05/2016.

BRAZIL. Ministry of Health. National Health Foundation. **Politica nacional de atençâo à saù dos povos indigenas**. 2 ed. Brasilia:

MS/FUNASA, 2002.

BRAZIL. Ministry of Health. National Oral Health Coordination. 3rd **National Oral Health Conference**: final report. Brasilia, 2004. 148p. Available at: http://portalsaude.saude.gov.br/ Accessed on 21/05/2016.

GIL, Antonio Carlos. **Methods and techniques of social research**. 6. ed. - Sao Paulo: Atlas, 2008.

HIROOKA, Lucila Brandao. **Oral health conditions in mother-child pairs in the indigenous population of the Middle and Lower Xingu**: dental caries and need for treatment. 2010. Available at: http://www.teses.usp.br/teses/disponiveis/17/17139/tde-02122010-091906/en-br.php Accessed on 29/04/2016.

MEDEIROS, Urubatan Vieira; ABREU, Carla Maria W. Protocol for oral health promotion in companies. **Brazilian Journal of Dentistry**. Vol.2, n°23, 2006. Available at:

http://bases.bireme.br/cgi-bin/wxislind.exe/iah/online/?IsisScript=iah/iah.xis&src=google&base=BBO&lang=p&nextAction=lnk&exprSearch=23316&indexSearch=I   D Accessed on 12/04/2016.

MOURA, Alice Bezerra de Mello. **The national health care policy for indigenous peoples**.   2012. Available at:

http://www.ufpe.br/remdipe/index.php?option=com   content&view=article&id=395&Itemid=251 Accessed on 14/04/32016.

SOUZA, Tiago Araùjo Coelho de; FERREIRA, Efigênia Ferreira e. Oral health among the Wajapi indigenous people of the state of Amapà. **Revista Tempus Actas de Saùde Coletiva**, V.6, n1, 2012. Available at: http://www.tempus.unb.br/index.php/tempus/article/view/1104 Accessed on 20/05/2016.

6. THE CONTRIBUTION OF NURSING IN THE CONTROL OF SELF-MEDICATION IN THE INDIGENOUS VILLAGE

Evaldo Silva do Nascimento, Clovis Luciano Giacomet.

INTRODUCTION

Self-medication is a problem that causes concern in the health sector, since the use of medicines without a doctor's prescription can relieve symptoms of illnesses, masking them and sometimes delaying diagnosis.

According to the World Health Organization (WHO) (2006), between 1995 and 2000, the sale and consumption of medicines grew significantly, especially in high-income countries. In 2000, total sales reached US$ 316 billion, of which US$ 33.9 billion were purchased without a doctor's prescription. In the same year, Brazil ranked ninth among the world's ten largest drug markets, with a value of US$ 5.2 billion.

Diehl and Grassi (2010) attribute this often abusive use of medicines to the impact of advertising on consumption and the high investments made by pharmaceutical companies in medicines that don't necessarily need a doctor's prescription, coupled with the fact that people find it difficult to access free medical care, often opting for self-medication.

There is also the cultural issue of the various social groups that make up Brazilian society, in which, not infrequently, alternative treatments are used with the use of "natural medicine", practiced by people who have no specific training, who have learned from their ancestors how to manipulate herbs that are said to cure various ailments (MENÉNDEZ, 2003).

Among these social groups are the indigenous populations, where the problem of the use of both prescribed and non-prescribed medication, as well as medication used on the basis of the knowledge of the *karai* (the person in charge of caring for the sick in the village), needs to be constantly monitored, since the indiscriminate use of medication is on the increase.

In view of this context, a concern about the subject arose and we decided to carry out this research, with the aim of verifying the use of self-medication in indigenous populations and its consequences in the lives of these individuals.

As there are few studies in Brazil, we chose to develop this work with indigenous peoples, because we have seen that nursing in general is not prepared to face this challenge, and urgent measures are needed so that this control is as early as possible, with this practice we will be providing a low consumption of industrialized or non-industrialized drugs.

Given that the rampant use of medicines among the indigenous population is notorious, it was necessary to look more deeply into how the drug reaches the individual and how they behave towards the nursing team that dispenses the drug.

It is important to remember that the medication is distributed to the indigenous client according to the doctor's note and the nurse's note when possible, but the biggest aggravation observed is that the medication is not being consumed properly in the home environment.

The role of nurses in controlling self-medication in an indigenous village. Defining the role of nurses in indigenous communities, identifying ways to control self-medication in indigenous communities and discussing the importance of the control and dispensation of medicines by nurses in indigenous villages.

THE INDIGENOUS POPULATION IN BRAZIL

Today, from an indigenous population estimated at 5 million at the time of the colonization of Brazil, there are only 897,000 Indians living in all Brazilian states, with the exception of Piaui and Rio Grande do Norte, divided into around 305 peoples, speaking 274 different languages, occupying around 12% of the Brazilian territory, a portion of whom live in urban regions, usually on the outskirts (IBGE, 2010).

Also according to FUNASA (2002), many of these peoples are threatened with disappearance, and some of them are in danger of biological reproduction, such is the reduction in population, as is the case in the state of Rondônia, where intense logging, mining and farming activities have caused high mortality rates, with an estimated population of 6.284 people in 1999, remnants of 22 peoples, is one example of this. While some of these societies are undergoing a process of population recovery, like the Pakaas Novos, for example, who now number more than 2,000, others, like the Latundê, are undergoing a process of reduction and currently number only 37 people.

INDIGENOUS HEALTH IN BRAZIL

According to FUNASA (2002), since the beginning of Portuguese colonization, indigenous people were cared for by missionaries in an integrated way with government policies.

At the beginning of the 20th century, with territorial and economic expansion, which brought with it the construction of railroad and telegraph lines, there were numerous massacres of indigenous peoples and a huge rise in mortality rates from communicable diseases, This led to the creation, in 1910, of the Service for the Protection of Indians and National Workers, which was attached to the Ministry of Agriculture and whose aim was to protect the Indians and progressively integrate their lands into the national production system.

However, the indigenous people were still seen as individuals in evolution, considered to be at an infantile stage of humanity and the assistance provided was sporadic and disorganized, limited to emergency or "pacifist" actions.

This situation lasted until the 1950s, with no public policies aimed at systematized care, which resulted in many deaths from infectious diseases that affected the indigenous populations, until the Air Sanitary Units Service was created, which aimed to bring health actions to populations in areas that were difficult to access, essentially focused on vaccination, dental care, tuberculosis control and other communicable diseases (BRASIL, 2002).

In 1967, the Service for the Protection of Indians and National Workers was abolished and FUNAI and the Volante Health Teams were created, which provided sporadic assistance to the indigenous communities in their area of coverage, providing medical care, administering vaccinations and supervising the work of the health personnel in these localities, who were reduced to nursing assistants and attendants.

However, this service went into decline after the financial crisis that hit Brazil in the 1970s, causing resources for care to become scarce, making the services provided even more precarious, in addition to the extinction of the Volante Health Teams, which ended up dissolving due to a lack of professionals who ended up settling in urban centers and in administrative activities, turning to a model of emergency and palliative care, provided by people with little qualification.

It is noteworthy that none of the initiatives related to the care of indigenous populations took into account the specificity of this population, ignoring their values, representations and practices related to health and illness, demonstrating disrespect for the context of the indigenous individual's relations with society and the environment in which they lived.

The situation described has only changed since the 1988 Constitution, which "stipulated the recognition and respect of the socio-cultural organizations of indigenous peoples, assuring them full civil capacity - making the institution of guardianship obsolete - and established the exclusive competence of the Union to legislate and deal with indigenous issues" (BRASIL, 2002).

The Constitution also defined the general principles of the Unified Health System (SUS), later regulated by Law 8.080/90, and established that the sole direction and responsibility for the federal management of the system lies with the Ministry of Health.

From then on, discussions took place in order to structure a system capable of offering more effective and punctual health care to the indigenous population, as was the case with the First National Conference for the Protection of Indigenous Health and the Second National Conference on Health for Indigenous Peoples, which took place in 1986 and 1993 respectively, on the recommendation of the Eighth and Ninth National Health Conferences. These two Conferences proposed the structuring of a differentiated model of care, based on the strategy of Special Indigenous Health Districts, as a way of guaranteeing indigenous peoples the right to universal and comprehensive access to health, meeting the needs perceived by the communities and involving the indigenous population in all stages of the process of planning, executing and evaluating actions (BRASIL, 2002).

In 1991, as part of the actions guided by the above-mentioned Conferences, by means of a decree, the government transferred responsibility for coordinating health actions aimed at indigenous populations to the Ministry of Health, establishing the Special Indigenous Health Districts as the basis for organizing health services. The Ministry of Health then created the Coordination of Indigenous Health (COSAI), which was responsible for implementing a new model of indigenous health care (BRASIL, 2002).

On October 17, 2007, FUNASA issued the controversial Ordinance No. 2.656, which regulated the Incentives for Basic and Specialized Care for Indigenous Peoples, revoking Ordinance No. 1.633/GM of September 14, 1999.

This decree sparked large demonstrations by indigenous peoples, dissatisfied with the policy that FUNASA was managing, who demanded the creation of a policy model compatible with the Arouca Law and the guidelines of the Second National Conference on Indigenous Health. As well as strengthening FUNASA, the ordinance opened up concrete prospects for the municipalization of indigenous health, exactly the opposite of what the indigenous peoples wanted.

It was only in August 2008, after constant demonstrations by the indigenous movement against FUNASA, and countless accusations of corruption and neglect in the execution of actions and services in indigenous areas, which had been generating overwhelming infant mortality and the spread of diseases, that the Minister of Health decided to listen to the complaints and proposals of the indigenous peoples.

After two years of waiting, the government issued Provisional Measure No. 483, which was approved by Congress and transformed into Law No. 12.314/2010. On October 19, 2010, Decree No. 7.336/2010 was issued, making official the creation of the Special Secretariat for Indigenous Health (SESAI).

This period of transition for the implementation of the new management of indigenous health was characterized by shared management between SESAI and FUNASA, and despite the government having set a deadline of three months for detailing its structure and other measures to make it operational, the situation dragged on for more than three years while health care in the communities went through critical moments.

At the end of 2012, the Articulation of Indigenous Peoples of Brazil (APIB) published a letter to the Minister of Health expressing the growing outcry of indigenous leaders, communities and organizations from all over Brazil, and their indignation at the worrying state of chaos and calamity in which indigenous health care has become, in conditions similar to those at the time of the management of the National Health Foundation (FUNASA). The document called for an effective intervention in SESAI so that it could actually fulfil its mission, in accordance with the expectations placed in it since its creation as a result of the struggle of Brazil's indigenous peoples and organizations.

SELF-MEDICATION

According to Silva, Goulart and Lazarini (2014), self-medication is the practice of taking medication without the advice and monitoring of a qualified health professional, i.e. taking medication at the risk of the person taking it.

These authors point out that this practice is quite common, regardless of the cultural level, economic or social position of the individuals and also the historical context involved, with the aim of relieving simple and recurring symptoms.

However, Masson, Lazarini and Conterno (2012) warn that even though this is a common practice and is understood and considered to be a form of self-care, it can become potentially dangerous to health, bearing in mind that no medication goes unnoticed by the body and can cause damage ranging from mild to serious.

Becker (2010) says that, looking at the historical context of self-medication, it is possible to see that the roots of this practice come from indigenous culture and black slaves, who used medicinal herbs, benzeduras and "spiritual cures" to treat the ailments that affected people. Thus, the author states that during the first four centuries of

Brazil's history, this was the practice that permeated the health care of mainly Indian and black slaves and farm employees, while the nobles sought medical treatment in Europe.

Nowadays, although these practices are almost extinct, self-medication has taken over, given the huge number of drug options on the market that don't require a doctor's prescription. According to ABIFARMA (Brazilian Association of Pharmaceutical Industries), around 20,000 people die every year in Brazil as a result of self-medication (SILVA; GOULART; LAZARINI, 2014).

Lessa and Bochner (2008) state that the indiscriminate use of medicines has become one of the major difficulties facing the health sector worldwide, mainly because the people who adopt this practice are unaware of the harm the medicine can cause, and it is identified as one of the biggest causes of human poisoning.

Ferreira, *et.al.* (2005), state that another risk factor is the quantity and variety of medicines that people have at home, referring to a veritable "therapeutic arsenal", which favors the practice of self-medication and, presenting as risks, accidental ingestion, causing intoxication, especially by children, in addition to losing effectiveness due to poor storage or even expired medicines.

Beckhauser, Valgas and Galato (2012) cite research by Fernandes (2000) which showed that in Porto Alegre, 97% of the households surveyed had at least one medicine in stock and the number of these ranged from one to eighty-nine items (with an average of 20 items), of which around 55% were purchased without a doctor's prescription and, of this total, 25% were expired and 24% were still being used.

From the above, it can be seen that self-medication is a serious health problem that can cause a lot of harm to the population, mainly due to their lack of knowledge about the risks of this practice.

SELF-MEDICATION IN INDIGENOUS POPULATIONS

With regard to self-medication by indigenous populations, the literature on the subject is scarce. Only three references on the subject were found.

In the study by Diehl and Grassi (2010), carried out in a Guarani village in the state of Santa Catarina, it was found that 236 consultations were carried out over a period of 103 days, with 458 medicines being prescribed, including analgesics, antibacterials, anthelmintics, anti-inflammatories, anti-rheumatic drugs and cough syrups. These were included in the National List of Essential Medicines (RENAME).

With regard to the medicines found during the home visits, which were carried out in 20 homes, an average of 2 to 5 medicines were found, with 10 different medicines being found in two homes and some with expired expiry dates, which caused concern among the health team accompanying the research. However, all the medicines had a doctor's prescription, since they were provided by a mobile health team that works directly in the village and the residents don't usually leave it.

The researchers also observed that the most frequent complaints were coughs, flu and diarrhea, and that the medicines found in the homes were mostly for these ailments.

In this research, the strong cultural influence of the presence of the *Karai*, a kind of "doctor" in the village, who is sought out before looking for health services, was reported. If the Karai tells him to look for a doctor, the indigenous person goes; if not, benzeduras and herbal teas are used to cure various ailments. The *Karai* also diagnose whether the illness is bodily or spiritual, demonstrating the strong link, even in places of strong acculturation, with the oldest traditions of the village, which sometimes proves to be an obstacle to medical treatment for various illnesses.

In this study, in particular, the number of people who practice self-medication was not considered relevant, emphasizing the care of the health teams that monitor the population and take care of this aspect.

In Souza's research (2007), it was found that the coexistence of the indigenous people with the medicines prescribed by doctors and those prepared by the village elders (usually the shaman), occurs relatively peacefully, with both being used.

However, the cultural issue has a lot to do with it, as once again the "bad spirits" are cited to explain many illnesses, and there is no need, according to the indigenous people, for a "doctor's" medicine, just to receive a blessing from the shaman and take a "garrafada", produced by boiling the bark, leaves, fruit and seeds of plants, adding a little sugar or honey, or by tanning the plants in cachaça.

Another important aspect observed by Souza (2007) was the question of how medicines are seen by indigenous people. They have a positive view, in the sense that medicines act quickly to relieve symptoms, and the negative view is linked to the danger they see in taking more than one medicine at the same time. They often don't take two or more medicines when prescribed by the doctor for fear that they might do harm, saving them for another occasion, which can lead to self-medication in other illness situations.

It is worth noting that the medication must currently be dispensed by the team by means of a note in the outpatient medical record, with the date and time of the prescription. What is observed among professionals in the field, especially in the village, is that this medication is mistakenly consumed at home by the recipient of the drug.

Most of these medicines were prescribed by the doctor who makes up the multidisciplinary team that serves the village and it was observed that, of the total found, 6.6% had no medical prescription, and it was not reported who "prescribed" the medication.

It was also found that 13.2% of the medicines had expired.

Based on the data collected and the interviews carried out by the authors, they came to the conclusion that the indigenous people sought medical attention, received the medication at the village health center and started the treatment, but when they didn't see its immediate effectiveness, they stopped the treatment and kept it, opting instead for traditional medicine, i.e. medicine made from the bush, usually guided by the village healer (DIEHL; ALMEIDA, 2012).

It is noteworthy that no references were found regarding indigenous people who leave the villages to sell handicrafts and spend periods away from them, which opens up space for the use of medicines without the knowledge of the health team that attends to them.

Nursing, especially in the indigenous area, plays a very important role in guiding these patients, informing them of the eminent risks of indiscriminate use of medication. It should also be remembered that nursing needs to put into practice the five rights of medication (right dose, right time, right medication, right route and right patient), so that we have a beneficial result in the promotion and recovery of the individual.

CONCLUSION

The use of self-medication in indigenous populations and its consequences in the lives of these individuals.

After the studies carried out, it was found that health care for indigenous people is provided by the Ministry of Health through the National Health Foundation, specifically in indigenous villages throughout the country, following a protocol established by the Special Secretariat for Indigenous Health (SESAI).

Medical and nursing consultations are usually carried out within the village itself and the prescription of medicines is made by the doctor of the multidisciplinary team that serves the village. These medicines are purchased at the health center and dispensed by the nurse and nursing technicians to the patients.

The research showed that many prescribed medicines are not used, because the culture of herbal medicine and blessings is still very present, and many medicines are stored and ingested later, without medical attention.

Affirming the above context, changes in a population's behavior depend on our attitudes as members of the Multidisciplinary Indigenous Health Team (EMSI). In view of the above, it is necessary for nurses to be prepared to work with health education, with the aim of making the indigenous population aware not to use medicines that are not officially prescribed by the doctor or nurse at the local Basic Health Unit (UBS).

The rates of self-medication reported in the surveys are relatively low, but no reference was found to indigenous people who spend time outside the village to sell their handicrafts, so the initial concern persists, prompting a structured field survey to obtain the relevant information.

The main purpose of this research was to focus on the contribution of nursing in the control and dispensation of drugs in the village, since this research needs to be more in-depth so that we have more concrete results on the indiscriminate use of drugs with indigenous villagers.

REFERENCES

BECKER, C. B. **Slaves and their relationship with the history of health on the southern border of Rio Grande do Sul in the 19th century**. X State History Meeting. BRAZIL IN THE SOUTH. July 26-30, 2010. Santa Maria - RS, Federal University of Santa Maria. Available at:

http://www.eeh2010.anpuhrs.org.br/resources/anais/9/1278786544
ARQUIVO_artigoanpuhoriginal.pdf Accessed on 17/02/2016.

BRAZIL. National Health Foundation. **National Policy for the Health Care of Indigenous Peoples**. - 2. ed. Brasilia: Ministry of Health. National Health Foundation, 2002.

DIEHL, E. E.; ALMEIDA, L. K. de. Medicines in a local indigenous context: the Xokleng "home pharmacy", Santa Catarina. **Revista de Antropologia Social dos Alunos do PPGAS-UFSCar**, v.4, n.1, jan.-jun., p.189-206, 2012. Available at: http://www.rau.ufscar.br/wp-content/uploads/2015/05/vol4no1_11_.DiehlAlmeida.pdf Accessed on 15/03/2016.

DIEHL, E. E.; GRASSI, F. Use of medicines in a Guaranido village on the coast of Santa Catarina, Brazil. **Cadernos de Saùde Pùblica**, Rio de Janeiro, 26(8):1549-1560, Aug, 2010. Available at: http://www.scielosp.org/pdf/csp/v26n8/09.pdf Accessed on 03/03/2016.

FERNANDES, L.C. Characterization and analysis of the home pharmacy or home stock of medicines. Dissertation (Master's Degree). Porto Alegre: Faculty of Pharmacy, UFRGS, 2000. In: Beckhauser, Gabriela C.; VALGAS, Cleidson; GALATO, Dayani. Profile of the household stock of medicines in homes with children. **Revista de Ciências Farmacêuticas Bàsica e Aplicada**. 2012. Available at: http://serv-bib.fcfar.unesp.br/seer/index.php/Cien_Farm/article/viewFile/2240/1_336 Accessed on 02/03/2016.

FERREIRA, W. A.; SILVA, M. E. S. T.; PAULA, A. C. C. F. F. de; RESENDE, C. de A. M. B.; Evaluation of Home Pharmacy in the Municipality of Divinopolis (MG) by Students of the Pharmacy Course at Unifenas. **Revista Infarma**, v.17, n° 7/9, 2005. Available at: http://www.cff.org.br/sistemas/geral/revista/pdf/19ZinfQ10.pdf Accessed on 23/02/2016.

IBGE - BRAZILIAN INSTITUTE OF GEOGRAPHY AND Statistics. **Indigenous census 2010**. 2010. Available at: http://indigenas.ibge.gov.br/ Accessed on 14/02/2016.

LESSA, M. de A.; BOCHNER, R. Analysis of hospital admissions of children under one year of age related to drug intoxication and adverse effects in Brazil. **Revista Brasileira de Epidemiologia**, v.11, n.4, p.660-674, 2008. Available at: http://www.scielo.br/scielo.php?script=sci arttext&pid=S1415- 790X2008000400013 Accessed on 23/02/2016.

MASSON, W.; FURTADO, P. L.; LAZARINI, C. A.; CONTERNO, L. de O. Self-medication among medical students at the Marilia Medical School, São Paulo. **Brazilian Journal of Health Research**. Vitória, 14(4): 82-89, Oct-Dec, 2012. Available at: http://periodicos.ufes.br/RBPS/article/view/5123 Accessed on 17/02/2016.

MENÉNDEZ, E. L. Models of disease care: from theoretical exclusions to practical articulations. **Ciênc. saùde coletiva vol.8 no.1 Rio de Janeiro 2003**. Available at: http://www.scielo.br/scielo.php?script=sci arttext&pid=S1413- 81232003000100014 Accessed on 12/02/2016.

WHO - WORLD HEALTH ORGANIZATION. **WHO policy perspectives on medicines**. Geneva, 2006. Available at: http://www.who.int/whr/2006/06 overview pr.pdf?ua=1 Accessed on 12/02/2016.

SILVA, F. M. da; GOULART, F. C.; LAZARINI, C. A. Characterization of the practice of self-medication and associated factors among university Nursing students. **Revista Eletrônica de Enfermagem**. [Internet]. 2014 Jul/Sep;16(3):644-51. Available at: https://www.fen.ufg.br/fen revista/v16/n3/pdf/v16n3a20.pdf Accessed on 17/02/2016.

SOUZA, L. C. de. Remédios do Mato and Remédios de Farmàcia: relações entre o sistema mèdico Fulni-ô e o sistema oficial de saù.

In: BRAZIL. Ministry of Health. **Traditional Indigenous Medicine in Context** - Proceedings of the First Monitoring Meeting. Luciane Ouriques Ferreira and Patricia Silva Osório (eds.). Vigisus II/Funasa Project. Brasilia: National Health Foundation, 2007. Available at: http://sis.funasa.gov.br/portal/publicacoes/pub1466.pdf Accessed on 12/03/2016.

7. DENTAL CARIES IN INDIGENOUS POPULATIONS OF BRAZIL: AN APPROACH TO IMPROVING ORAL HEALTH

Kelly Barboza Ribeiro, Clóvis Luciano Giacomet

Introduction

The World Health Organization (WHO) states that oral diseases, such as dental caries and periodontal disease, have become a global health problem in both industrialized and developing countries, especially in poor communities[1].

Because it is more frequent, caries has been intensively studied from an etiological and epidemiological point of view, with the aim of better understanding its determinants, prevalence and distribution, as well as establishing preventive measures[2]. Epidemiology provides the basis for analyzing the distribution and magnitude of health problems in the population[3].

The verification of decayed, missing and filled teeth (DMFT index) in oral health epidemiological surveys is the most accepted and recommended by the WHO for different age groups and especially for school-aged children[4]. The organization establishes the age of 12 as the basic parameter for the indicator, with the following severity scale: very low prevalence (0.1-1.1); low prevalence (1.2-2.6); moderate prevalence (2.7-4.4); and high prevalence (4.5-6.5)[5].

The WHO recently joined forces with the International Dental Federation (IDF) and the International Association for Dental Research (IADR) to announce the 2020 goals for dental caries[6,7,8]. In this document, entitled "*Global Goals for Oral Health*", it is stated that 80% of children aged 6 should be free of cavities and by the age of 12 the DMFT index should be less than 1.5 by the year 2020.[6,7]

In Brazil, the first national survey carried out in 16 state capitals in 1986 showed a DMFT at the age of 12 of 6.7. In 2003, the first oral health survey was carried out, which included, in addition to all 27 capitals, the inland municipalities of the five regions, a survey that became known as Projeto Brasil 2003. In this study, the DMFT at the age of 12 was 2.78. In 2010, the SBBRASIL 2010 Project was carried out and, in this 2010 survey, the DMFT at the age of 12 was 2.07, corresponding to a reduction of 26.2% in 7 years[9].

However, there are significant regional differences. When comparing the country's regions, the differences in average DMFT at 12 years of age are significant: the North (with 3.16), the Northeast (with 2.63) and also the Midwest (with 2.63) are worse off than the Southeast (1.72) and South (2.06)[9].

On the other hand, the oral health conditions of the indigenous population are little known in Brazil. The available studies point to a high prevalence of dental caries among indigenous people and a worsening trend[9,10], which is a serious public health problem and highlights the social exclusion of these groups[12].

Therefore, the questions that arise are: (i) what is the importance of knowing the rate of tooth decay in order to improve the oral health of indigenous populations, (ii) what is the incidence of tooth decay in indigenous communities; (iii) what is the role of the dentist in preventing oral diseases, and (iv) what is the importance of preventing tooth decay in indigenous people?

The dentist is considered to play a fundamental role in the prevention of oral diseases, since he or she carries out a survey of individual needs, socio-economic conditions and the level of understanding of oral hygiene. They establish action strategies, implement promotion and prevention programs and provide collective and individual dental care to all individuals in the community. [23]

The incidence of tooth decay in indigenous communities is high and is thought to be related to socio-economic, cultural and biological factors, as well as the limitations of the oral health programs implemented by the public authorities since then.

Contact with the non-indigenous population has brought about a change in dietary patterns, including the intake of industrialized and carbohydrate-rich foods in their diet. The importance of preventing tooth decay in indigenous people goes hand in hand with a better physical and emotional quality of life. Prevention reduces the risk of the disease and/or its recurrence and is also the most economical way of caring for oral health. It raises awareness of the need for hygiene habits and self-care to maintain good health.

The aim of this study is to understand dental caries in indigenous populations. To this end, the role of the dentist in the prevention of oral diseases will be described, identifying the incidence of caries in indigenous communities and discussing the importance of caries prevention in indigenous people. The qualitative factors analyzed in this study are epidemiology, tooth decay, indigenous populations and oral health.

DENTAL CARIES IN INDIGENOUS POPULATIONS IN BRAZIL

For dental caries, the CPO index by Klein and Palmer (1937) is known worldwide, as it fulfills the necessary requirements in terms of reliability, as well as being easy to apply. The CPO-D index (decayed, missing or filled permanent teeth) measures the experience of decay in permanent teeth. This index is an average resulting from the total number of decayed permanent teeth plus filled and missing permanent teeth, divided by the number of individuals examined in a given population. [22]

Knowledge of the dental caries index of a given population is relevant to public health, since it enables the presence and severity of this pathology to be detected, thus allowing public policies to be applied with focus and objectivity to solve the health problems identified.

In indigenous oral health, the document Guidelines for Oral Health Care in the DSEI presents a model of health care that takes into account the epidemiological reality, as a fundamental point to help local managers establish standards of measures for oral health/disease. [23]

The development of research into dental caries in recent decades has led to a better understanding of the process by which the disease develops, as well as the possibility of controlling its onset and progression in its earliest stages. In this sense, dentistry is no longer just about surgery and restoration, but also about prevention and health promotion.[24]

In this sense, this study is justified by the need for knowledge about the epidemiological situation of dental caries in indigenous groups in Brazil to enable the implementation of more efficient oral health policies and actions. The oral health conditions, measured by the DMFT index, of 07 indigenous groups from different regions of the country will be presented: Wajapi (Amapà / North region); Xakriabà (Minas Gerais / Southeast region); Baniwa (Amazonas / North region); Xavante (Mato Grosso / Center West region); Xingu (Mato Grosso / Center West region) and Xukuru and Ororubà (Pernambuco / Northeast region). No studies on the prevalence of dental caries in indigenous populations in the South were found in the literature.

According to the 2010 IBGE census, there are currently 817,963 indigenous people in Brazil, representing 305 different ethnic groups and 274 languages. This contingent inhabits all the states of the federation, including the Federal District[14] .

Demographic information on the indigenous peoples served by the Indigenous Health Subsystem, through SESAI, shows that in 2013, 655,111 indigenous people were registered in the Indigenous Health Care Information System (SIASI). This population was distributed in 4,702 villages, within or outside the boundaries of 615 indigenous lands, covering 467 Brazilian municipalities. In the same year, the distribution of the indigenous population by Brazilian region was 46.9% in the North, 25.2% in the Northeast, 17.6% in the Midwest and 10.3% in the South-Southeast.[26]

The rapprochement with non-indigenous society, the emergence of paid activities in the villages, the presence of non-indigenous professionals, who bring large quantities of food with them for their stay in the indigenous area, has led to changes in the diet and influenced the increased consumption of industrialized foods[15] . They also traditionally eat a diet rich in starch (manioc, corn). This type of diet is closely related to the onset of tooth decay. The bacteria present in the oral cavity ferment the residues of starches and carbohydrates, transforming them into acids, mainly lactic acid, which demineralizes the dental tissues, resulting in lesions.

In this context, the epidemiological profile of oral health in the indigenous population presents worrying data.

In a survey of dental needs carried out with the Wajâpi population, by the oral health team of the Special Indigenous Health District (DSEI) of Amapà and Northern Parà, in partnership with Non-Governmental Organizations (NGOs), in 2003, it was found that 73,2% of the population surveyed immediately needed multiple restorative and/or surgical procedures and the average DMFT at 12 years of age was 3.7[15] , higher than the average of 3.1 reported by the Ministry of Health (SB Brazil Project 2003) for the general population of the northern region at the same age .[15,16]

Among the indigenous schoolchildren from the Xakriabà reserve, located in the municipality of Sâo Joao das Missoes, in the north of the state of Minas Gerais, among the children attended by the Sumaré and Brejo Mata Fome base centers and the Rancharia village, only the Brejo Mata Fome and Rancharia base centers met the WHO target for the age of 12. However, there was no statistically significant difference between the three villages studied. The fact that the 12-year-old target was met may be related to fluoride toothbrushing. It is therefore necessary to distribute fluoridated toothbrushes and toothpastes to all the Xakriabàs. A high-impact, low-cost and very effective initiative[17] .

In a study carried out in 2004, the Baniwa Indians of Alto Rio Negro, Amazonas, had an average DMFT of 6.0 in the 12-14 age group. The dental actions carried out by the DSEI Alto Rio Negro teams, based in São Gabriel da Cachoeira, included two visits a year by the dental team to each community, where they distributed a tube of fluoridated dentifrice and a toothbrush per resident, as well as individual clinical consultations, health education activities and supervised brushing. The water used for consumption came from the Içana River and was not artificially fluoridated. The staple diet continues to be manioc and its derivatives, wild fruits, fish and game, but industrialized foods are already part of everyday life, even serving as barter items, or when they have a source of income they use part of it to buy this type of food[18] .

A study carried out among the Xavantes of Etenheritipa between 1999 and 2009, coordinated by Arantes, evaluated the impacts of the implementation of an oral health program in partnership between the Indigenous Association and a non-governmental organization, based on educational, preventive and assistance components.

The educational component sought to incorporate self-care habits by building new concepts about health and disease. The preventive component provided regular access to fluoride, either through toothpaste or topical application. And the care component, dental care, pain relief, removal of foci of infection, restorations of recoverable teeth and basic periodontal therapy.

In the period between 2004 and 2007, there was a reduction in tooth decay levels for the 11-15 age group, compared to the average values in 2004. According to the study, the reduction was mainly due to prevention activities[12,19].

Also through partnerships between public institutions and non-governmental organizations, an Oral Health Program was carried out in the Xingu Indigenous Park (Middle and Lower Xingu) based on the diagnosis of local needs, taking into account the demographic and epidemiological profile, the historical and cultural context and the recognition of local leaders[19,20]. The effectiveness of this program in the region was later proven through an epidemiological survey from 2001 to 2006, indicating a reduction in the DMFT index between the ages of 12 and 34 anos [19,21].

A study carried out in the state of Pernambuco with the Xukuru de Ororubà ethnic group aimed to analyze the oral health condition of this population aged between 10 and 14 years. Oral examinations revealed an average DMFT index of 2.38. At the index age of 12, considered to be the international standard for comparability, the DMFT had an average of 2.73. Of all the individuals examined, 26.61% were free of decay[25].

However, if this percentage (26.61%) is compared with the index presented by SBBrasil 2010 (which includes the general population), it is much lower, creating a picture of inequality between the two populations (indigenous and non-indigenous).

When we analyze the data presented, we see that there are differences in DMFT indices between the different ethnic groups and also with non-indigenous people. While some communities reap the rewards of successfully implemented oral health programs, others receive visits every six months, leaving the population unattended.

Of all the public policies aimed at improving the health conditions of a population, one of the most important is related to the food that will make up the diet, since it is associated with various chronic diseases such as diabetes mellitus, hypertension, cardiovascular diseases and tooth decay. Of the components of the diet, sugar is one of the most common and is one of the main etiological factors of tooth decay.[27]

Public policies relating to oral hygiene, smoking, health services and especially the use of fluoride are also extremely important.[27]

It is clear that health services are fundamental to the oral health of the community. However, the predominance of the care approach must be questioned. Changes are therefore needed in the traditional ways in which dental professionals work, so that health actions are redirected towards the field of prevention and health promotion.[13]

In dentistry, much has been done to solve the problems caused by tooth decay and periodontal disease. However, it is known that it is much easier to prevent the onset of these diseases than it is to treat them once they have set in or even to limit the extent of their damage. [28]

In this sense, the oral health team is an integral and important part of the population's health, since the National Oral Health Policy - Smiling Brazil - proposes the Incorporation of health promotion and protection actions, such as fluoridation of water supplies, health education, supervised dental hygiene and topical fluoride applications. With the exception of water fluoridation, the other actions are directly related to the role of the dental surgeon as an actor in this process.[27]

As with the family health strategy (ESF), the work of the oral health team in indigenous health aims, among other things, to carry out collective and individual procedures in places where there are no dental practices, to carry out integrated actions with other areas of health and to use other social spaces to develop collective oral health actions, as well as to encourage a shift from individual to collective care. [23]

In order for the indigenous health dentist to fulfill his role efficiently, it is essential to know the characteristics of the population's epidemiological profile, not only in terms of the most prevalent diseases, but also the socio-economic conditions of the community, their habits, customs and lifestyle and their health needs - felt or not, including by extension the infrastructure of available services. In this way, the professional will be able to better identify the main groups of health promotion, protection and recovery actions to be developed as a priority. [27]

It is clear that dentists have a fundamental role to play in preventing oral diseases, especially tooth decay. Because he has a broad view of the health-disease process, he must be able to understand people, taking into account their individual needs and not just a set of signs and symptoms restricted to the oral cavity. They must balance prevention and cure[13] . And by identifying the problems of different population groups, they can establish action strategies, implementing targeted programs for collective dental promotion and prevention.

In order to achieve success in preventing dental caries among indigenous peoples, and consequently change the epidemiological scenario, it is essential that the indigenous oral health program - Brasil Sorridente Indigena (launched by SESAI in 2011) - is strongly focused, not only on increasing the indigenous population's access to dental care, but primarily on actions to prevent and promote oral health in the villages.

Conclusion

Thus, indigenous populations have a greater experience of dental caries than the general Brazilian population. The change in the dietary pattern experienced by indigenous peoples, together with the lack of guidance on oral hygiene, the absence of exposure to fluoride - especially in its systemic form - as well as the difficulty of access by the indigenous population to the oral health services of the Indigenous Health Subsystem can be considered explanatory factors for the current epidemiological picture.

In this context, the oral health teams of the Special Indigenous Health Districts (DSEI) play a central role in tackling tooth decay, especially in relation to the challenge of implementing health promotion programs built on knowledge of the reality and local specificities and based on strategic and interconnected pillars: normativity (pacts, agreements, norms), education, assistance, prevention and behavior change.

Bibliography:

1- WORLD HEALTH ORGANIZATION. **WHO releases new report on global problem of oral diseases**. Geneva: WHO; 2004.

2- PINTO, *V.* G. **Oral Health. International Overview. Brasilia: National Secretariat for Special Health Programs**. Ministry of Health, 1990.

3- ALMEIDA, T.F. et al. **Oral health conditions in children, adolescents and adults registered in Family Health units in the Municipality of Salvador, State of Bahia, Brazil, in 2005**.Epidemiol. Serv. Saùde, Brasilia, v. 21; n.1; p.109-118, jan-mar 2012.

4- PRADO, J.S.; et al. **Dental condition and oral hygiene habits in school-aged children**. Rev. Biociênc. Taubaté, v.7; n.1; p.63-69, jan-jun2001.

5- INTERAGENCY NETWORK OF INFORMATION FOR HEALTH (RIPSA): **Basic indicators for health in Brazil: concepts and applications**. RIPASA- 2. ed. - Brasilia: Pan American Health Organization, 2008. 349 p.: ill

6- BARATA, C.; VEIGA, N.; MENDES, C.; ARAUJO, F.; RIBEIRO, O.; COELHO, I.; **Determination of DMFT and oral health behaviors in a sample of adolescents from the municipality of Mangual** Rev. Port. Stomatol. Med. Dent. Cir. Maxillofacial. 54; n.1; p.27-32, jan-mar 2013.

7- PETERSEN, P. E.; **Priorities for research for oral health in the 21st Century - the approach of the WHO Global Oral Health Programme**. Community Dent Health. v.22; n.2; p.71-74, jun 2005.

8- HOBDELL, M.; PETERSEN, P. E.; CLARKSON, J.; JOHNSON, N. **Global goals for oral health 2020**.Int. Dent. J. v.53; n.5; p.285-288, oct 2005.

9- BRAZIL. MINISTRY OF HEALTH. **SBBrasil Project 2010: National Oral Health Survey - Main Results**. Brasilia-DF, 2011.

10- ARANTES, R.; SANTOS, R.V.; COIMBRA JR, C.E.A. **Oral health in the Xavante indigenous population of Pimentel Barbosa, Mato Grosso, Brazil.** Cad Saùde Pùblica2001; 17:375-384.

11-ARANTES, R. **Oral health of indigenous peoples in Brazil: current panorama and perspectives**. In: Coimbra Jr. CEA, Santos RV, Escobar AL, organizers. *Epidemiology and health of indigenous peoples in Brazil.* Rio de Janeiro: Fiocruz/ABRASCO; 2003. p. 4972.

12- ARANTES, R. **Oral health of the indigenous peoples of Brazil and the case of the Xavante of Mato Grosso.** Doctoral thesis presented to the Sérgio Arouca National School of Public Health. Rio de Janeiro: s.n., 2005.

13- AERTS, D., ABEGG, C., CESA, K.. **The role of the dental surgeon** in the Unified Health System. Ciência & Saùde Coletiva, 9(1):131-138, 2004.

14- BRAZIL. Ministry of Justice. National Indian Foundation. Indians of Brazil. www.funai.gov.br (accessed 26/April/2016).

15- SOUZA, T. A. C., FERREIRA, E,. **Oral health among the Wajâpi indigenous people of the state of Amapà**. Tempus Actas de Saùde Coletiva journal

16- BRAZIL. Ministry of Health. Secretariat of Health Care, Department of Primary Health Care. **SB Brasil 2003 Project: oral health conditions of the Brazilian population 2002-2003: main results. Brasilia; 2004**.

17- **Adyler Duarte Diab**. Dental caries in Xakriabà indigenous children. Faculty of Health Sciences, University of Brasilia, Brasilia-DF, Brazil **Simone Dutra Lucas (Advisor)** Faculty of Health Sciences, University of Brasilia, Brasilia-DF, Brazil

18- CARNEIRO, M. C. G., SANTOS, R. V., GARNELO, L., REBELO, M. A. B., CIMBRA JR. C. **Dental caries and the need for dental treatment among the Baniwa Indians of the Upper Rio Negro, Amazonas.** Ciênc. saùde coletiva vol.13 no.6 Rio de Janeiro Nov./Dec. 2008

19- ARANTES, R., PAULO, F. **Dental caries among indigenous peoples in Brazil: implications for oral health programs.** Electronic journal TEMPUS Acta. v. 7, n. 4 (2013)

20-Lemos P. N., HIROOKA, L. B., NUNES, S. A. C., ARANTES, R., MESTRINER, S. F., MESTRINER, W. Jr. **The oral health care model in the Middle and Lower Xingu: partnerships, processes and perspectives.** Ciência e Saùde coletiva; 2010;15(Suppl. 1):1449- 1456.

21-PACAGNELLA, R. C. **Epidemiological profile of oral health in the Xingu Indigenous Park between 2001 and 2006**. Master's dissertation. Ribeirao Preto Medical School/USP, 2007.

22- PIGOZZO, M. N., LAGANA, D. C. CAMPO, T. N., YAMADA, M. C.

M. **The importance of indices in clinical dental research: a literature review**. Revista de Odontologia da Universidade Cidade de Sao Paulo 2008 Sep-Dec; 20(3): 280-7

23- - BRAZIL. Guidelines **for Oral Health Care in the DSEI**. National Health Foundation, 2007.

24- DIAS A. A. **Saúde bucal coletiva metodologia de trabalho e pràticas**. Sâo Paulo: Santos; 2006.

25- MAURICIO, H. A., MORERIRA, R. S. **Oral health conditions of the Xukuru do Ororubà ethnic group in Pernambuco: multilevel analysis.** REV BRAS EPIDEMIOL JUL-SET 2014; 787-800.

26- - BRAZIL. Ministry of Health. Special Secretariat for Indigenous Health.   Link: http://portalsaude.saude.gov.br/index.php/o-ministerio/principal/secretarias/secretaria-sesai/mais-sobre-   sesai/9518-destaques

27- BRAZIL. Coordination of Oral Health, Department of Primary Care, Secretariat of Health Care, Ministry of Health. **National oral health policy. Brasilia: Ministry of Health**; 2004.

28- SANTOS, P. A, RODRIGUES, J. A., GARCIA, P. P. N. S **Knowledge about cavity and periodontal disease prevention and oral hygiene behavior of elementary school teachers.** Cienc. Odontol. Bras. 2003 jan./mar.; 6 (1): 67-74.

8. THE INCLUSION OF INDIGENOUS PEOPLES THROUGH EDUCATION AND WORK: AN APPROACH TO IMPROVING QUALITY OF LIFE

Luzemar das Graças Borges, Clóvis Luciano Giacomet

INTRODUCTION

The inclusion of indigenous peoples through education and work has been a subject of reflection and anxiety for educators at all levels of education, as it presupposes changes in representations about the subjects to be included and the identities of all those involved in the process.

The process of inclusion of indigenous peoples through education and work has been happening slowly, but has been well received by both indigenous peoples and society in general.

We start from the idea that the word inclusion suggests the perfect insertion of the individual into an environment in a participatory way that is sufficient to develop their human potential, making them capable of taking advantage of possible opportunities for themselves and for society. Satisfactory inclusion presupposes socio-economic, political, emotional and cultural factors.

When they enter school, indigenous people bring with them their life history, which has a strong influence on their learning process. It will therefore be of great importance how they are welcomed by the school and how they remain in the school environment in order to ensure their full development and thus have more job opportunities.

From a research perspective, this paper seeks to respond to a need that has arisen in relation to the quality of life and recognition of an entire ethnic group. Through a bibliographical study, it seeks to clarify how this process takes place, with the aim of describing how indigenous peoples are integrated through education and work, how they behave and how they are received by the members of the ordinary school community.

By investigating reality in a harmonious but concise way, it is clear that everyone needs to become aware of the need to integrate indigenous people into society.

Priority is given to the need to include indigenous people, but there needs to be a major change in the means that involve this need, serving as a phase for today's society to look for ways to alleviate this problem.

The debates on the inclusion of indigenous peoples through education and work reveal data that is even more important at this time of affirmation of the practices and theories that underpin it.

Talking about this new reality for these people means understanding that their development and socialization can be quite satisfactory when they come to be seen as individuals capable of being part of a world made up of skilled and competent people.

The aim of this study is to see how indigenous peoples are integrated through education and work,

Characterizing indigenous ethnic groups, describing indigenous protection and legalization, determining the conditions of indigenous work.

CHARACTERIZATION OF INDIGENOUS ETHNIC GROUPS

We can see that there are various types of indigenous ethnic groups, but we must first understand what ethnicity means and that each ethnic group has its own way of relating to work.

According to Brasil (1996), the term ethnicity is used in anthropological studies to differentiate social groups in the context of the social sciences.

However, the word best fits the term ethnic community, which has a conceptual category of analysis and participates in a community, constructing itself socially, existing, problematizing, articulating the isolation of people in the communications of the differences they appropriate, establishing ethnic boundaries. The term ethnic group is generally used in anthropological literature to designate a community that: 1) to a large extent biologically self-perpetuating; 2) shares fundamental cultural values manifestly realized in cultural forms; 3) integrates a field of communication and interaction; 4) counts as members who identify themselves [sic], and, are identified by others and who constitute a category distinguishable from other categories of the same order (Barth, 1976).

If we understand what ethnicity is, we can conclude that it is part of all ethnic categories, classifying the interaction of normative behavior of ethnic groups as an emphasis.

An ethnic group can be operationally defined as a collectivity of people who participate in certain patterns of normative behavior; they are part of a larger population, interacting with people from other collectivities, within a global social system. The term ethnicity refers to the degree to which members of the collectivity conform to these norms of participation in the course of social interaction (BARTH, 1976, apud SILVA, 1986).

Ethnicity means the interaction of ethnic groups based on a social context, the point being that ethnicity has visible cultural or racial characteristics and is defined by an ethnic group.

In relation to the Indians, they are ethnic groups more identified by their cultural traits, always in the same way, with a lot of similarity between them.

PROTECTION AND LEGALIZATION OF INDIGENOUS CULTURE

The 1988 Constitution was a milestone in the conquest of indigenous rights, due to the greater participation and autonomy acquired by indigenous descendants in the construction of the country and to the fact that various rights were protected.

They went through a historical moment of recognition as a people distinguished by their social organization and no longer just by their connection to natural goods that could be enjoyed by society.

To understand the importance of consolidating these rights in a Magna Carta is to realize that almost always when we talk about Indians, we also talk about conflicts and domination. In colonial Brazil, the Indians were usually related to a single ethnic group and most of the time they were kept close only by economic interests, which always represented a great delay in the guarantees of indigenous rights.

Until then, the legislation had catered to the colonizers, and the improvements that could be applied to the Indians remained on an imaginary level. Used as labor, their lands were incorporated into those of the province and many villages ceased to exist.

In Araùjo's (2006) work, important information is obtained, such as the fact that in the first Brazilian Constitution, from 1824 to 1967, there were no important mentions of indigenous rights, which went on for decades without due attention, mainly due to the lack of importance given to the issue by the ruling classes of the time.

Still in his book, Araùjo (2006) mentions that the draft of the first Constitution (1824) alluded to the catechesis and civilization of the Indians, but the Constitution didn't even mention the subject. Only the 1934 Constitution addressed the issue of indigenous land rights and their integration into society, and these issues were presented in the following constitutions.

INDIGENOUS WORK

With regard to work, there are many distinctions and prejudices against many races, but especially the indigenous, and the racial issue in Brazil has been placed at the center of the social policy agenda.

Over time, there has been an increase in inclusion and training policies for them, so that they can improve the quality of life in their communities. FUNAI trains indigenous professionals through courses offered by public and private bodies and non-governmental organizations. The intention is to train the individual so that they can help their own tribesmen gain access to education and health, and to help researchers in a wide variety of fields, especially linguistics and education (Brasil, 2010).

As a result of this work, the indigenous public's interest in gaining more knowledge has grown dramatically, and social policies have begun to explicitly promote their integration into the labor market.

The 2010 Census indicated that 52.9% of indigenous people had no income whatsoever, an even higher proportion in rural areas (65.7%). However, several factors make it difficult to obtain information on the income of indigenous workers: many jobs are done collectively, leisure and work are not easily separated and the relationship with the land has enormous significance, without the notion of private property. Income analysis indicates differentiated relationships between indigenous people and work (BRASIL, IBGE. Censo 2010).

The aim is not to get them out of their villages, but to give them the conditions to be able to work there, in the village, and with that, having more knowledge, improve the quality of life of the Indians who live there.

This includes so many universalist policies that apply to the entire indigenous population, and they have quotas to enter because of their race, and there are many who specialize and have become Indians, doctors, teachers and even government secretaries.

The development of such policies varies widely, but together they seek to address a wide range of social exclusions that manifest themselves economically, psychologically, politically and culturally. This change is a milestone in Brazilian racial thinking, as important as the earlier ideological transition from white supremacy to racial democracy.

WORKING CONDITIONS OF INDIANS IN TODAY'S SOCIETY

Some Indians have their work recognized, they are part of the labor market, but their numbers are minimal, and the majority suffer exploitation in relation to their work, with many being recruited to work in sugarcane fields, in sugarcane mills, having to work endless hours and receiving a much lower wage than other workers, according to information in the Jornal de São Paulo on July 21, 2008.

However, what is perceived in society in general is the classification of the indigenous person as someone who doesn't like to work, who is only satisfied with what they fish and hunt, but it is known that this is no longer the case today, with the indigenous person increasingly seeking the job market and making their rights prevail, trying to insert themselves into this market that is still so "closed" to them.

INDIGENOUS ETHNIC GROUPS AND EDUCATION

The conquest of the rights of indigenous peoples is the realization of their educational rights, won through the demands of the indigenous movement in the Federal Constitution of 1988, in the Law of Guidelines and Bases of National Education (LDB), of 1996, and in the National Education Plan (PNE) of 2001, which represented the emergence of a new concept of the indigenous school, characterized as a community, intercultural, bilingual/multilingual, specific and differentiated school.

Within this new perspective in which the indigenous school has been conceptualized and implemented in recent years, indigenous school education cannot be thought of outside the specific contexts of indigenous education in each community.

Indigenous Education refers to all the educational processes used by each indigenous people to teach activities, whether complex or mundane (MAHER, 2006).

According to the author, in indigenous societies, traditional teachings occur spontaneously, daily and continuously, without a specific space or subject for teaching and learning.

INDIGENOUS PEOPLE IN THE SCHOOL ENVIRONMENT

Indigenous people in the school environment are part of educational processes that go through the same traditional teachings, spontaneously, daily and continuously, leaving room for the knowledge of the specific subject to teach and learn.

The school is the entire physical space of the community [...]. In indigenous education, there is no such thing as a "teacher". There are several teachers for the child. The mother teaches; she is a teacher. The father is a teacher, the old man is a teacher, the uncle is a teacher, the older brother is a teacher... and everyone is a pupil. As in our society, there is no single "holder of knowledge" authorized by an institution to educate children and young people (MAHER, 2006).

Thus, there is a differentiation between the teachings of the indigenous people and the other races, and it is from this differentiation that a harmonious way of understanding and establishing goals and precepts between human beings is sought.

CONCLUSION

Considering education as the knowledge of the construction of language, in terms of encouragement that leads to the recognition that all races are equal before justice and also in terms of the benefits they should have, each with its own characteristics, alienating care with the search to transform coexistence ever better.

For indigenous people too, all learning processes take place as each child or adult develops on their own within a set of relationships with others, being autonomous but thinking of the greater good. Their educational practices give them the opportunity to see themselves as members of a whole, integrators and creators. This coexistence with the other, implying a spontaneous transformation, exists to the extent that the other is accepted as legitimate in his or her difference, in other words, openness to otherness and the abandonment of coercive and domineering actions.

Learning in indigenous communities here is collective, and for that to happen they need learners who can guarantee the dialog of their knowledge and their transformation as people. Thus, the role of the school in the lives of indigenous people means that this learning takes place in a continuous process, from the perspective that one learns by living with others. Valuing knowledge is based on self-knowledge, in other words, on the ability to experience what you say and for your speech to be an expression of what you feel, making you feel like an integral part of the community.

And the work also plays an important role in the growth of the indigenous person as a person who is searching for their own path and makes the actions and reactions that take place in their daily lives more visible.

REFERENCES

ARAÙJO, A. V. **Povos Indigenas e As Leis dos Brancos**: Direito à Diferença. Brasilia: Ministry of Education, Secretariat for Continuing Education, Literacy and Diversity. Rio de Janeiro: LACED/National Museum, 2006.

BARTH,F. (org.) **Los Grupos Étnicos y Sus Fronteras.** Mexico City: Fondo de Cultura Económica, 1976. Translation: Maria Tereza Pàdua.

BRAZIL. Brazilian Institute of Geography and Statistics (IBGE). **Census 2010**. Available at: <http://censo2010.ibge.gov.br/noticiascenso?view=noticia&id=1¬icia=2194&t=censo-2010-populacaoindigena-896-9-mil-tem-305-etnias-fala-274>. Accessed on: 20/03/2016.

MAHER, T. M. Indigenous Teacher Training: An Introductory Discussion. In: GRUPIONI, Luiz Donisete Benzi (Org.). **Formação de professores indigenas**: repensando trajetórias. Brasilia: Ministry of Education, Department of Continuing Education, Literacy and Diversity, 2006.

SILVA, B. (coord.) **Dicionârio de Ciências Sociais.** Rio de Janeiro: FGV, 1986.

9. THE NURSE AND DIFFERENTIATED CARE FOR INDIGENOUS SOCIETIES

Paula Regina Jensen, Clovis Luciano Giacomet

INTRODUCTION

According to data from FUNAI (2013) - the National Indian Foundation, the current indigenous population in Brazil is made up of 490,000 people, belonging to 220 peoples who speak more than 180 languages. Based on this diversity, each of these peoples is organized in different ways and also has different ways of conceiving the health-disease process and the therapeutic interventions adopted when necessary.

In an effort to provide differentiated care for these populations, since August 1999, the Ministry of Health, through FUNASA - the National Health Foundation, has taken on the responsibility of structuring care for indigenous populations, with the creation of the National Policy for the Health Care of Indigenous Peoples, an integral part of the National Health Policy, which provides for the right of these populations to differentiated care by the Unified Health System - SUS - while respecting the cultural specificities of each indigenous people.

The Indigenous Health Subsystem of the Unified Health System (SUS) is organized into 34 Special Indigenous Health Districts - DSEI. It is a dynamic ethnic-cultural, geographic, population and administrative space that is well delimited and has no direct relationship with the boundaries of the states and municipalities where the indigenous lands are located (BRASIL, 2013).

As you can see, the public authorities, through FUNAI and the Ministry of Health, are trying to offer differentiated care to the indigenous population, since the specific characteristics of these peoples require care geared towards their conditions, their culture, in short, their way of life.

In view of Brazilian legislation which, through Law No. 9.836 of September 23, 1999, art. 19 F, provides for health care to be provided to indigenous populations, which must "take into account the local reality and the specificities of the culture of indigenous peoples and the model to be adopted for indigenous health care, which must be based on a differentiated and global approach, taking into account the aspects of health care" (BRASIL, 1999), it is necessary to acquire knowledge that can deal with this care in an effective way, and this is what this research project aims to do.

The integrative literature review was used to develop the study, whose guiding question was: "What evidence is available in the literature on differentiated health care for indigenous populations?"

The inclusion criteria were works that were related to the objective of the study, which was differentiated health care for indigenous populations. Thus, articles written only in Portuguese were selected, in full, from 2000 to 2014, using BIREME (Virtual Health Library) as sources for consultation, using as descriptors indigenous populations, differentiated care for indigenous populations, health-disease process.

As for the exclusion criteria, we looked at works that were not in line with the established objectives, that were not in their entirety, published in a language other than Portuguese, material of unknown origin, non-scientific and that were not in the period mentioned in the inclusion criteria.

The general objective of the research was to verify how health care is provided to indigenous populations and, as specific objectives, to trace the trajectory of health care for indigenous populations in Brazil; to clarify the understanding of the health-disease process in general and for indigenous people; emphasize the importance of the work of nursing professionals in providing differentiated care to indigenous populations;

highlight the need for humanized care in providing care to indigenous populations and; clarify the need for and importance of differentiated care for indigenous populations.

From this perspective, and given that the researcher works directly with indigenous communities, I was interested in highlighting the importance of nurses' work with these populations, as well as the peculiarities of this work.

UNDERSTANDING THE HEALTH-DISEASE PROCESS

According to Câmara (et.al., 2012), although various concepts of the health-disease process have been established, over time these concepts have been transformed according to the different ways in which society exists, which is constantly changing with the acquisition of new knowledge and the transformation of its culture and forms of organization.

The understanding of both health and illness depends on one's understanding of the relationships established with the environment in which one lives, which can vary according to the place, culture and historical moment in which one lives.

According to Vianna (2012), "illness cannot be understood only by means of pathophysiological measurements, because what establishes the state of illness is suffering, pain, pleasure, in short, the values and feelings expressed by the subjective body that falls ill".

Meanwhile, the World Health Organization defines health as "a state of complete physical, mental and social well-being and not merely the absence of disease and infirmity". Most authors on the subject criticize this definition, since the complete balance between physical, mental and social well-being in the turbulent times in which society currently lives sounds like a utopia (SEGRE; FERRAZ, 1997).

Brêtas and Gamba (2006) consider that:

[...] for health, it is necessary to start from the dimension of being, because it is there that the definitions of normal or pathological occur. What is considered normal in one individual may not be in another; there is no rigidity in the process. In this way, we can deduce that human beings need to know themselves, they need to be able to evaluate the transformations their bodies undergo and identify the signs they express. This process is only feasible from a relational perspective, since the normal and the pathological can only be appreciated in a relationship.

Thus, Vianna (2012) argues that for a more complete view of the health-disease process, it is necessary to take into account the distinction between disease as defined by care systems and health as perceived by individuals, also including the dimension of well-being in a broader sense.

For Brêtas and Gambà (2006):

[...] health and illness are not two sides of the same coin. In fact, if we consider a health system such as the SUS, it is possible to see that actions aimed at diagnosing and treating diseases are only two of its activities. Social inclusion, promoting equity or visibility and citizenship are considered health actions. The understanding of health as a relatively autonomous social device in relation to the idea of illness, and the repercussions that this new understanding brings to social life and everyday practices in general and health services in particular, opens up new possibilities in the conception of the health and illness process.

As you can see, the understanding of the health-disease process varies according to people's conceptions of the time, culture and region.

UNDERSTANDING THE HEALTH-DISEASE PROCESS

FOR THE INDIGENOUS

In the research carried out by Silva, Gonçalves and Lopes Neto (2003), in two indigenous villages in Amazonas, with the aim of verifying the indigenous people's understanding of the health-disease process, the authors were able to see that the indigenous people did not understand the seriousness of certain health problems, nor did they establish links between the disease and its causes, which the researchers attributed to the lack of sanitation, hygiene and preventive actions.

Fracolli and Bertolozzi (2001) consider that the understanding of "[...] health/disease is directly linked to the way in which human beings, in the course of their existence, have appropriated nature in order to transform it, seeking to meet their needs".

The indigenous people, despite already having a fairly advanced culture, still have their own beliefs and way of life, making it difficult for them to learn about the disease and its causes, as well as forms of prevention and treatment.

In this sense, Langdon (2000) states that "it is essential to respect the notions, values and expectations of each ethnic group".

In this respect, it is important to emphasize that the principle of the National Policy for the Health Care of Indigenous Peoples preaches "[...] respect for the conceptions, values and practices relating to the health/disease process specific to each indigenous society" (BRASIL, 2002).

In a study carried out by Lazarotto and Baratieri (et.al., 2007), it became clear that, of the 132 Kaingàng families who took part, the majority based their beliefs about health/disease on their own indigenous culture and that customs and beliefs are also linked to the search for the most important figure in the village, the shaman. It is based on his opinion that they seek treatment at the health unit.

Analyzing the results of this research, it can be seen that, although they have medical assistance, the belief in the "diagnosis" of the shaman is still predominant and it is on his advice that they go to seek help at the medical clinic, making it clear that respect for the values of each ethnic group must be considered, as advised by the National Policy on Health Care for Indigenous Peoples (LAZAROTTO; BARATIERI, *et.al.*, 2007).

In the research by Pellon and Vargas (2010), carried out in three villages in Espirito Santo, it became clear that the perceptions of the indigenous people also take into account the ethnic values of their culture, since, according to these authors: Cultural practice recommends that the disease be diagnosed within the *opy* (prayer house) by the *Karai* (shaman) who should indicate the appropriate treatment, not depriving himself of referring the patient to the public health care system if he deems it necessary.

However, Pellon and Vargas (2007) cite in their research the dissatisfaction of indigenous people with the type of care provided in health units due to the prejudice and ethnocentrism shown by some professionals, which leads them to avoid seeking health care, making it clear that:

[...] the ways in which discrimination is expressed are not always so obvious, because they are often subliminally embedded in the webs of social and economic relationships that structure and determine the expression of the health-disease process, both in its direct and indirect determinants. However, experiencing discrimination can in itself be a trigger for illness and becomes more serious when the experience takes place within health care services, as it can generate strong emotions, ranging from fear and mistrust to anger and frustration, compromising

This shows that indigenous people's understanding of the health-disease process is linked to their cultural and ethnic perceptions and values, and that differentiated care for this community is essential because of these peculiarities.

THE HEALTH OF INDIGENOUS PEOPLES: ADVANCES AND SETBACKS

According to FUNASA (2002), since the beginning of Portuguese colonization, the indigenous people were cared for by the missionaries in an integrated way with government policies.

At the beginning of the 20th century, with territorial and economic expansion, which brought with it the construction of railroad and telegraph lines, there were numerous massacres of indigenous peoples and a huge rise in mortality rates from communicable diseases, This led to the creation, in 1910, of the Service for the Protection of Indians and National Workers, which was attached to the Ministry of Agriculture and whose aim was to protect the Indians and progressively integrate their lands into the national production system.

However, the indigenous people were still seen as individuals in evolution, considered to be at an infantile stage of humanity and the assistance provided was sporadic and disorganized, limited to emergency or "pacifist" actions.

This situation lasted until the 1950s, with no public policies aimed at systematized care, which resulted in many deaths from infectious and contagious diseases that affected the indigenous populations, until the creation of the Air Sanitary Units Service, which aimed to bring health actions to the populations of areas that were difficult to access, essentially focused on vaccination, dental care, tuberculosis control and other communicable diseases. (BRAZIL, 2002).

In 1967, the Service for the Protection of Indians and National Workers was abolished and FUNAI and the Volante Health Teams were created, which provided sporadic assistance to the indigenous communities in their area of coverage, providing medical care, administering vaccinations and supervising the work of the health personnel in these locations, who were limited to nursing assistants and attendants.

However, this service fell into decline after the financial crisis that hit Brazil in the 1970s, causing resources for care to become scarce, further compromising the services provided, in addition to the extinction of the Volante Health Teams, which ended up dissolving due to a lack of professionals who ended up settling in urban centers and in administrative activities, turning to a model of emergency and palliative care, provided by people with little qualification.

It is noteworthy that none of the initiatives related to the care of indigenous populations took into account the specificity of this population, ignoring their values, representations and practices related to health and illness, demonstrating disrespect for the context of the indigenous individual's relationship with society and the environment in which they lived.

The situation described only changed with the 1988 Constitution, which "stipulated the recognition and respect of the socio-cultural organizations of indigenous peoples, assuring them full civil capacity - making the institution of guardianship obsolete - and established the exclusive competence of the Union to legislate and deal with indigenous issues" (BRASIL, 2002).

This Constitution also defined the general principles of the Unified Health System (SUS), later regulated by Law 8.080/90, and established that the sole direction and responsibility for the federal management of the system lies with the Ministry of Health.

From then on, discussions took place in order to structure a system capable of offering more effective and timely health care to the indigenous population, as was the case with the First National Conference on the Protection of Indigenous Health and the Second National Conference on Health for Indigenous Peoples, which took place in 1986 and 1993 respectively, on the recommendation of the Eighth and Ninth National Health Conferences.

These two Conferences proposed the structuring of a differentiated model of care, based on the strategy of Special Indigenous Health Districts, as a way of guaranteeing indigenous peoples the right to universal and comprehensive access to health, meeting the needs perceived by the communities and involving the indigenous population in all stages of the process of planning, executing and evaluating actions (BRASIL, 2002).

In 1991, as part of the actions guided by the above-mentioned Conferences, by means of a decree, the government transferred responsibility for coordinating health actions aimed at indigenous populations to the Ministry of Health, establishing the Special Indigenous Health Districts as the basis for organizing health services. The Ministry of Health then created the Coordination of Indigenous Health (COSAI), which was responsible for implementing a new model of indigenous health care (BRASIL, 2002).

In the same year, Resolution 11, of October 13, 1991, of the National Health Council (CNS), created the Inter-Sectoral Commission on Indigenous Health (CISI), whose main task was to advise the CNS on the development of principles and guidelines for government policies in the field of indigenous health.

However, in 1994, also by means of a presidential decree, the coordination of health actions was returned to FUNAI, delegating to it the responsibility for recovering the health of sick indigenous people and prevention to the Ministry of Health, which would be responsible for immunization, sanitation, human resources training and endemic disease control (BRASIL, 2002).

This defragmentation of the indigenous health care model meant that responsibility was divided between FUNASA and FUNAI, causing a "breakdown" in the care provided to the populations, since the actions were disconnected and individual (BRASIL, 2002).

In 1997, the Inter-Sectoral Commission on Indigenous Health of the National Health Council (CISI/CNS) requested the intervention of the Federal Public Prosecutor's Office (6- CCR/MPF) because of the federal government's failure to implement an adequate policy for indigenous health care.

The public hearing held in November 1997 concluded that the responsibility established in the Federal Constitution for indigenous health care lay with the Ministry of Health at the federal level, and that "the refusal of institutions linked to the SUS to provide this assistance constituted an illegal act that could be confronted through the competent channels" (ALTINI, et.al., 2013).

As a result of the increased pressure, in 1999 the federal government issued Decree No. 3.156 and promoted the approval of the "Arouca Law" (Law No. 9.836, of September 23, 1999) in the National Congress. This law was written by Congressman Sérgio Arouca, one of the leaders of the Health Reform, regulating the guidelines approved at the Second National Conference on Indigenous Health, and had been shelved in the National Congress since 1994 (BRASIL, 2002).

Indigenous health policy became the exclusive responsibility of the

Ministry of Health: "The Ministry of Health will establish the policies and guidelines for the promotion, prevention and recovery of indigenous health, whose actions will be carried out by FUNASA". The Arouca Law ordered the federal government to set up the Indigenous Health Care Subsystem (SASI-SUS), based on the Special Indigenous Health Districts (DSEIs). The 34 DSEIs were then created through Ordinance 852/1999 (ALTINI, et.al, 2013).

In view of the serious health problems faced by indigenous peoples, in 1999 the federal government sanctioned Law No. 9.836, adding provisions to Law No. 8.080 of 1990, laying down the conditions for the promotion, protection and recovery of health, the organization and functioning of the corresponding services in relation to indigenous populations, establishing, at that time, the Indigenous Health Care Subsystem, which is linked to the Department of Indigenous Health Care.

[...] the mission of planning, coordinating and supervising comprehensive health care activities for indigenous peoples; guiding and supporting the implementation of health care programs for the indigenous population, according to SUS guidelines; planning, coordinating and supervising health education activities in the Special Indigenous Sanitary Districts; coordinating the preparation of norms and guidelines for the operationalization of health care actions in the Special Indigenous Sanitary Districts; providing technical advice to the teams of the Special Indigenous Sanitary Districts in the development of health care actions; support the preparation of District Indigenous Health Plans and coordinate building and environmental sanitation actions within the Special Indigenous Sanitary Districts (MOURA, 2012).

According to Ministry of Health Ordinance No. 2607, of December 10, 2004, the Special Indigenous Health Districts are a model for organizing services, which include a set of technical activities, aimed at rationalized and qualified health care measures, promoting the reorganization of the health network and health practices and developing administrative-managerial activities necessary for the provision of care, with social control.

Also in 2009, the 34 Special Indigenous Health Districts (DSEIs) were given administrative autonomy. The DSEIs began to function as decentralized management units, responsible for health care and basic sanitation in each region. The autonomy of the districts reduces the bureaucracy of indigenous health care, which is now integrated and articulated with the entire Unified Health System (SUS) (BRASIL, 2002).

In 2004, through ordinances 69 and 70, FUNASA established new guidelines for indigenous health, with the aim of recovering direct execution and reducing the role of the contracted organizations, limiting them to hiring staff, providing care in the villages with supplies, transporting indigenous people from the villages, and buying fuel to make these journeys. In 2006, the Fòrum de Presidentes dos Conselhos Distritais de Saùde Indigena (Forum of Presidents of District Indigenous Health Councils) was set up to act in an advisory and propositional capacity, in line with the other decision-making bodies of the SUS (BRASIL, 2002). In the process of holding the fourth National Conference on Indigenous Health in 2006, several district conferences put forward the proposal to create the Special Secretariat for Indigenous Health (SESAI), due to the worsening of the recurring problems of poor management, authoritarianism, political use and corruption in FUNASA's regional coordinations and central bodies. This proposal was taken to the plenary of the national stage of the conference, and ended up being defeated by a small margin of votes, prompting the denunciation by a large part of the indigenous delegation of manipulation in the work of the conference (ALTINI, et.al, 2013).

On October 17, 2007, FUNASA issued the controversial Ordinance No. 2,656, which regulated the Incentives for Basic and Specialized Care for Indigenous Peoples, revoking Ordinance No. 1,633/GM of September 14, 1999.

This decree sparked large demonstrations by indigenous peoples, dissatisfied with the policy that FUNASA was managing, who demanded the creation of a policy model compatible with the Arouca Law and with the guidelines of the Second National Conference on Indigenous Health. As well as strengthening FUNASA, the ordinance opened up concrete prospects for the municipalization of indigenous health, exactly the opposite of what the indigenous peoples wanted (BRASIL, 2002).

It was only in August 2008, after constant demonstrations by the indigenous movement against FUNASA, and countless accusations of corruption and neglect in the execution of actions and services in indigenous areas, which had been generating overwhelming infant mortality and the spread of diseases, that the Minister of Health decided to listen to the complaints and proposals of the indigenous peoples (BRASIL, 2002).

During this same period, the Federal Court of Auditors (TCU) carried out an audit of FUNASA, focusing on issues relating to the management of indigenous health policy. At the same time, the Labor Court ruled that the federal government was responsible and therefore the manager of the health policy, and that outsourcing was an illegal practice (BRASIL, 2002).

At the end of 2008, Bill No. 3.958 was presented with a view to amending Law No. 10.683/2003, which deals with the organization of the Presidency of the Republic and the Ministries, and creating the Secretariat for Primary Care and Health Promotion, which would house indigenous health.

In the explanatory memorandum to this project, the Minister of Health proposed the transfer of Funasa's powers and responsibilities to this secretariat. Also as a result of pressure from indigenous peoples, a Working Group was set up with the participation of indigenous leaders (ordinances 3.034/2008 and 3.035/2008 - GAB/MS), whose aim was to discuss and present proposals, actions and measures to be implemented within the Ministry of Health, with regard to the management of health services offered to indigenous peoples (BRASIL, 2002).

After two years of waiting, the government issued Provisional Measure No. 483, which was approved by Congress and transformed into Law No. 12.314/2010. On October 19, 2010, Decree No. 7.336/2010 was issued, making official the creation of the Special Secretariat for Indigenous Health (SESAI).

This transitional period for the implementation of the new management of indigenous health was characterized by shared management between SESAI and FUNASA, and despite the government having set a deadline of three months for detailing its structure and other measures to make it operational, the situation dragged on for more than three years while health care in the communities went through critical moments (BRASIL, 2002).

At the end of 2012, the Articulation of Indigenous Peoples of Brazil (APIB) published a letter to the Minister of Health expressing the growing outcry of indigenous leaders, communities and organizations throughout Brazil, and their indignation at the worrying state of chaos and calamity in which indigenous health care has become, in conditions similar to those at the time of the management of the National Health Foundation (FUNASA).

The document called for an effective intervention in SESAI so that it could actually fulfil its mission, in accordance with the expectations placed in it since its creation, as a result of the struggle of Brazil's indigenous peoples and organizations (BRASIL, 2002).

Today, from an indigenous population estimated at 5 million at the time of the colonization of Brazil, there are only 370,000 Indians living in all Brazilian states, with the exception of Piaui and Rio Grande do Norte, divided into around 210 peoples, speaking 170 different languages, occupying around 12% of the Brazilian territory, a portion of whom live in urban areas, usually on the outskirts (BRASIL, 2002).

Also according to FUNASA (2002), many of these peoples are threatened with disappearance, and some of them are in danger of biological reproduction, such is the reduction in population, as is the case in the state of Rondônia, where intense logging, mining and farming activities have caused extremely high mortality rates, with an estimated population in 1999 of 6,284 people, remnants of 22 peoples, is one example of this. While some of these societies are undergoing a process of population recovery, like the Pakaas Novos, for example, who now number more than 2,000, others, like the Latundê,

have been reduced and currently have only 37 people.

Among the indigenous populations, the most frequent morbidities are acute respiratory and gastrointestinal infections, malaria, tuberculosis, sexually transmitted diseases, malnutrition and vaccine-preventable diseases, showing a health situation characterized by the high occurrence of illnesses that could be significantly reduced with the establishment of systematic and continuous basic health care actions within the indigenous areas (BRASIL, 2002).

In addition to these problems, in regions where the indigenous population maintains a closer relationship with the local population (which is increasingly common), health problems related to changes in the way of life, especially in diet, are appearing, usually causing hypertension, diabetes, cancer, alcoholism and depression, drawing attention to the frightening rise in the number of suicides in these populations (BRASIL, 2002).

THE WORK OF NURSING PROFESSIONALS IN THE DIFFERENTIATED CARE OF INDIGENOUS POPULATIONS

From its beginnings to the present day, nursing has undergone transformations as society and its demands have changed.

Defined as early as the 19th century by Florence Naghtingale as the "art of caring", albeit in a non-systematized way, today nursing can be defined as:

[...] an action or activity carried out predominantly by women, who need it to reproduce their own existence and use knowledge from other sciences and a synthesis produced by themselves to grasp the object of health in what concerns their specific field (nursing care?), envisioning the end product, which is to meet social needs, i.e. health promotion, disease prevention and the recovery of the individual or the control of the population's health (ALMEIDA; ROCHA, 1997).

These authors also emphasize that nursing is responsible, through care, for the comfort, reception and well-being of patients, whether providing care, coordinating other sectors to provide care and promoting patient autonomy through health education.

HUMANIZATION AS A REQUIREMENT FOR DIFFERENTIATED CARE

In nursing today, one of the most discussed topics is humanization, which according to Deslandes (2004) is represented by: a set of initiatives aimed at producing health care capable of reconciling the best available technology with the promotion of acceptance and ethical and cultural respect for the patient, work spaces that are conducive to good technical practice and the satisfaction of health professionals and users.

Thus, it is a challenge for the nursing team, which needs to master not only the technical aspect, but also the ethical and humanitarian aspect, in which caring goes beyond the scope of procedures, and also involves caring for the person as a being endowed with feelings and emotions.

Humanization in the health sector means going beyond the technical-scientific-political competence of the professionals. It involves developing competence in interpersonal relationships, which need to be based on respect for life, solidarity and sensitivity to perceiving the unique needs of the subjects involved (CASATE and CORRÊA, 2005).

From what the authors have said, it can be seen that humanization involves much more than just applying techniques and procedures, but seeing the other person in their entirety, as a human being with not only a physical aspect, but also emotional and psychological aspects, which need to be taken into account when aiming to humanize assistance and care.

Finally, Rolim and Cardoso (2006) conclude by saying that humanization is necessary, since the indiscriminate valorization of technological aspects, without taking into account subjectivity, solidarity, touch and human interaction, can result in assistance centered on the machine, the disease and not on the human being.

And nowadays in nursing care, this type of care is no longer conceivable, because the object of care is also made up of emotion, of feelings that need to be taken into account when caring.

Humanized care

Humanized care has been one of the most discussed aspects of nursing today, as it is no longer conceivable to only provide patients with technical and procedural care. The humanist vision, which seeks to respect the human being and consider them in their entirety, makes a real difference, because the existence of another being is perceived and praised, the other gives the sense of self. Caring for the other fosters caring for oneself, and the growth of one's own being results in caring for the being of the other. In short, it is an ethical attitude in which human beings perceive and recognize each other's rights (WALDOL, 2004).

Care involves responsibility, commitment, involvement with one's own being, with others and with the universe. In other words, the caregiver is involved, interacts and takes responsibility for the growth and well-being of the other, be it an idea, a plant, an animal or nature as a whole. It seeks to improve the nursing being, not just as a profession, but as a mission of care, i.e. not merely technical care, because there is a direct link with the human being involving their interpersonal relationship, transforming them into a professional of differentiated quality (WALDOL, 2004).

Humanization represents a set of initiatives aimed at producing health care that is capable of reconciling the best available technology with the promotion of a welcoming atmosphere, ethical and cultural respect for patients, work spaces that are conducive to good technical practice and the satisfaction of health professionals and users (DELANDES, 2004).

According to Moraes (2004),

Humanizing according to ethical values fundamentally consists of making a practice beautiful, no matter how much it deals with what is most degrading, painful and sad about human nature: Suffering, deterioration and death. It therefore refers to the possibility of assuming an ethical position of respect for others and of recognizing one's limits. The key point in the work of humanization lies in strengthening this ethical position of articulating scientific-technical care, already constructed, known and mastered, with care that incorporates the need, exploration and acceptance of the unpredictable, the uncontrollable, the indifferent and singular.

The authors thus explain the core of humanization, when they put scientific-technical care together with respect for others, their pain and their fragile condition in the face of illness.

Simoes, et.al. (2007) point out that:

Humanization is an expression that is difficult to conceptualize, given its subjective, complex and multidimensional nature. Inserted in the context of health, humanization, much more than the clinical quality of professionals, requires quality of behaviour. Portuguese dictionaries define the word humanize as: to make human, to civilize, to make human. It is therefore possible to say that humanization is a process that is constantly being transformed and is influenced by the context in which it takes place.

In this context, it can be inferred that humanization, so much discussed today, requires this attitude of being human, of putting oneself in the position of the other person and their family and of providing assistance in such a way that care goes beyond the frontier of technicality and mechanism, making care more effective and likely to be successful.

Vila and Rossi (2002) state that a:

[...] humanization must be part of the nursing philosophy. The physical environment, material and technological resources are no more significant than the human essence. This will guide the thinking and actions of the nursing team, especially the nurses, making them capable of criticizing and building a more humane reality (...).

These authors stress the importance of humanization, especially in the

ICU, where the environment seems more hostile and where nurses have a greater stress load, which can, according to them, lead to a certain "hardening" of the professional, who sometimes chooses to remain emotionally distant from the patient, mechanizing actions and, consequently, dehumanizing this relationship (VILA; ROSSI, 2002).

From a perspective of humanization, it is imperative that the nursing team is aware of its role, not only as a professional with technical training, but also that it develops this ability to humanize care, especially through communication, an essential element of this humanization process (BEDIN, et.al., 2004).

Corbani; Brêtas and Matheus (2009) point out that:

Nurses need to use their scientific knowledge and also their ability to observe and perceive. By acting in this way and planning, they will be able to visualize the patient's needs and understand their problems. The other professionals who provide care to patients can be efficient in their nursing procedures, but this is not enough to care; caring is more than that, it is natural.

From what the authors have said, it can be seen that humanized care is much more than simply applying techniques and procedures, but welcoming, understanding, guiding and giving oneself to those being cared for.

No matter how difficult it may be, no matter how challenging the day-to-day work may often be, professionals need to overcome these difficulties and carry out their work always bearing in mind the other person, their family and the situation they are going through, and thus, by putting themselves in the other person's shoes, this work will certainly be humanized.

DIFFERENTIATED CARE FOR INDIGENOUS POPULATIONS

According to Vianna (2012):

Working in indigenous health care in their own habitat has its peculiarities, which invariably brings difficulties for the professional, but also offers moments of profound learning for their professional work.

The author's words reflect the reality of professionals working with indigenous communities. In the research by Silva, Gonçalves and Lopes Neto, various difficulties were mentioned, such as long and tiring journeys that often have to be made on foot, adapting the work and the professional's conceptions to the local reality, the lack of suitable places to carry out the work, the itinerancy of some groups and, the greatest of all, the resistance of the indigenous people to receiving care, given their culture and belief, who often prefer to be attended only by the tribe's healer. This is in addition to the problem of communication between the nurse and the patient, which, as previously discussed, is one of the most important aspects of humanized care (VIANA, 2012).

Authors such as Diehl, Langdon and Dias-Scopel (2012) emphasize that there is no clear definition of differentiated care, and that in official documents, differentiated care is presented differently by the notions of "articulation", "integration" and "incorporation" of traditional practices.

The notions of integration and incorporation subject traditional practices to the determination of efficacy measured by biomedical epistemology, implying an instrumental fragmentation of indigenous health systems, selecting only those practices that have been scientifically proven (DIEHL; LANGDON; DIASSCOPEL, 2012).

Thus, in order to provide differentiated health care to indigenous populations, in 1999 the indigenous health agent (AIS) was institutionalized as part of the teams that provide primary care services in the villages, since, according to Diehl, Langdon and Dias-Scopel (2012):

Differentiated care includes respect for the conceptions, values and health practices of each people and articulation between indigenous and biomedical knowledge, and the indigenous agent is the mediator between this knowledge, as well as between the community and the team members.

The main activities of the Indigenous Health Agents are patient monitoring, care, first aid, prevention and health promotion. However, this work is not always carried out completely, as it depends on the degree of integration of the group and their understanding of the different nature of the work, success in offering services that respect and articulate with traditional practices depends very much on the commitment and efforts to train all members of the Multidisciplinary Teams of Primary Care for Indigenous Health, including the AIS, in differentiated care (DIEHL, LANGDON, DIAS-SCOPEL, 2012).

Training to care for indigenous populations from this perspective is of fundamental importance, since understanding the specificity of these people, their culture and their beliefs is fundamental to developing a satisfactory job, which is not an easy task, according to Langdon (1999).

[...] it is important that the training of professionals who deal with indigenous health devotes enough time for them to deeply understand the anthropological concept of relativism and also the concept of culture. They should be familiar with the nature of the indigenous health system, and how its practices are part of their culture as a symbolic system, made up of interrelated values, representations and meanings (LANGDON, 1999).

According to the author, many professionals who work with indigenous communities still carry a lot of prejudice towards them, hindering the effectiveness of health programs and actions.

[...] there is little evidence of mutual respect in the daily life of health services, which are characterized by hierarchical relationships and ignorance. In prevention and healing activities, it is common to hear health professionals expressing common prejudices about the Indians, characterizing or condemning them as dirty, ignorant of the concepts of health and illness, disobedient patients or resistant to treatment recommendations, and incapable of understanding them. In general, interventions in the health area are carried out without due respect for knowledge of the group's culture, and so professionals express ethnocentric attitudes and carry out their practices without recognizing how the cultural specificity of the group influences the success of their work (LANGDON, 1999).

It is clear from the author's speech that differentiated care is only possible once every professional working with indigenous communities understands the peculiarities of these people and respects them, seeking to understand and integrate into their way of life.

The National Policy for Indigenous Health Care, linked to the National Health Policy of the Ministry of Health, makes it clear that the training of human resources for indigenous health should be prioritized as a fundamental instrument for adapting the actions of SUS health professionals and services to the specificities of health care for indigenous peoples and to the new technical, legal, political and organizational realities of services.

However, it is essential that each professional is committed to the work to be carried out, in the sense of seeking different ways of integrating with the indigenous communities so that this differentiated service can be effective.

CONCLUSION

At the end of this research, it was found that although indigenous health is included in official documents, such as the 1988 Federal Constitution, and has public policies aimed at providing differentiated care, there is still a long way to go before it reaches the ideal and indigenous peoples can be cared for in such a way that their health is preserved.

The indigenous societies in Brazil currently number approximately 500,000 people, living in almost all Brazilian regions, distributed among 225 different tribes, making up 0.25% of the Brazilian population, in addition to those who live outside indigenous lands, including in urban areas.

Each of these peoples has a system of beliefs and values, despite the process of acculturation they have undergone over the years, which often distorts this system and generates situations of conflict and previously unknown situations, such as the frightening increase in the rate of suicide, violence and previously unreported diseases such as hypertension and diabetes, making health actions even more urgent in these communities.

It was also found that, for the indigenous people, the health-disease process is sometimes not understood, with illness being attributed to factors established by the culture, such as the action of "bad spirits", when, in fact, there is a lack of basic sanitation, hygiene and care to prevent illness. Most of the time, when an illness occurs, the village shaman is the first to be consulted and only if he advises it is a medical service sought. This situation makes it difficult for the health teams to act, as it is not always easy to reach them and convince them to seek care.

Another factor reported in the research exposed during this work is the unease that indigenous people feel when they are attended to in health units, as they often face the prejudice of some professionals who have no knowledge of the specificities that guide the lives of indigenous peoples, their way of being and thinking, often being classified as "vagabonds", "dirty" and "negligent".

Thus, it is clear that these populations need and have the right to differentiated care, which takes into account their perceptions of the health-disease process and values their culture, beliefs and values. We need professionals who have undergone training in the area and who are willing to listen, to seek integration with the indigenous communities, gaining their trust so that, when planning and implementing health actions, they can really be developed in a way that doesn't hurt the value system of each tribe, but that can promote disease prevention and health as a whole, not just in the physical aspect, but also in the social aspect.

Nursing professionals, who have closer contact with these populations, need to be sure that when they choose this job, they will encounter many difficulties and challenges, but that these can be overcome if they have a real interest in making a difference in caring for indigenous people.

It is worth pointing out that there is no clear concept of differentiated care for indigenous peoples, but with regard to the role of nursing in this context, the study carried out revealed that it consists of humanized care which prioritizes understanding and respect for the beliefs, values and culture of indigenous communities, within this premise, to carry out work that can improve the quality of life of these individuals who, after the arrival of the indigenous people in Brazil more than 500 years ago, went from being the owners of the land to marginalized individuals who seem to receive only crumbs of what was rightfully theirs.

Finally, at the beginning of this research, the aim was to highlight the importance of the role of nurses in providing differentiated health care to indigenous peoples and we conclude that this objective was achieved, hoping that more and more nursing professionals realize the need to really provide differentiated care, given that this is a differentiated population and that indigenous health is increasingly prioritized in Brazilian society.

REFERENCES

ALMEIDA, M. C. P. de; ROCHA, S. M. M. **O trabalho** de **enfermagem**. São Paulo: Cortez, 1997.

ALTINI, E.; RODRIGUES, G.; PADILHA, L.; MORAES, P. DI; LIEBGOTT, R. A. A **Politica de Atençâo à Saù Indigena no Brasil:** breve recuperaQăo histórica sobre a política de assistência à saúde nas comunidades indigenas. Indigenous Missionary Council: São Paulo, 2013. Available at: http://6ccr.pgr.mpf.mp.br/institucional/grupos-de trabalho/saude/cartilha-sobre-saude-indigena-cimi

BEDIN, E.; RIBEIRO, L. B. M.; BARRETO, R. A. S. S. Humanizaçâo da assistência de enfermagem em centro cirùrgico. **Revista Eletrônica de Enfermagem**, v. 06, n. 03, 2004. Available at: http://www.fen.ufg.br/revista/revista6_3/13_Revisao3.html

BRAZIL. National Health Foundation. **National Health**

Health Care for Indigenous Peoples. - 2. ed. Brasilia: Ministry of Health. National Health Foundation, 2002.

BRAZIL. **National Survey on Alcohol Consumption Patterns in the Brazilian Population**. National Anti-Drugs Secretariat, 2007. Available at:

http://bvsms.saude.gov.br/bvs/publicacoes/relatorio_padroes_consu mo_alcool.pdf

BRAZIL. Ministry of Health. National Health Foundation. **Politica nacional de atençâo à saù dos povos indigenas**. 2 ed. Brasilia: MS/FUNASA, 2002.

BRÊTAS, A. C. P.; GAMBA, M. A. **Enfermagem e saùde do adulto**.

Barueri: Manole, 2006.

CÂMARA, A. M. C. S.; MELO, V. L. C.; (et.al). Perception of the Health-Disease Process: Meanings and Values of Health Education. **Brazilian Journal of Medical Education**. 2012. Available at: http://www.scielo.br/pdf/rbem/v36n1s1/v36n1s1a06.pdf

CASATE, J. C.; CORREA, A. K. Humanization of health care: knowledge conveyed in the Brazilian nursing literature. **Latin American Journal of Nursing**. V. 13, n. 1, p. 105-111   , 2005. Available

em:http://www.scielo.br/scielo.php?pid=s010411692005000100017 &script=sci arttext

CORBANI, N. M. de S.; BRÊTAS, A. C. P.; MATHEUS, M. C. C. Humanization   of   nursing   care: what   is   it? **Brazilian Journal of**

enfermagem.   vol.62,   no.3,   Brasilia   Mai/Jun.   2009.Available at:http://www.scielo.br/scielo.php?pid=S003471672009000300003 &script=sci_arttext

DESLANDES, S. F.. Analysis of the official discourse on the humanization of hospital care. **Ciência & Saùde Coletiva**, 2004. 9(1):7-14. Available at: http://www.scielo.br/pdf/csc/v9n1/19819.pdf

DIEHL, E. E.; LANGDON, E. J.; DIAS-SCOPEL, R.I P.

Contribution of indigenous health workers to differentiated health care for Brazil's indigenous peoples. 2012.

Available at:

http://www.scielo.br/scielo.php?script=sci_arttext&pid=S0102-311X2012000500002

FRACOLI, L. A.; BERTOLOZZI, M. R. The approach to the health-disease process of family members and the collective. In: BRAZIL.

Institute for Health Development. University of São Paulo. Ministry of Health. Nursing manual. Brasilia: IDS/USP/MS, 2001.

FRAGA, T. F.; AMANTE, L. N.; ANDERS, J. C.; PADILHA, M. I. C. de S.; HENCKEMAEIR, b.; COSTA, R.; BOCK, L. F. Mothers' perception of the communication process in the neonatal intensive care unit. **Revista Eletrônica de Enfermagem**. [Internet]. 2009;11(3):612-9. Available at: http://www.fen.ufg.br/revista/v11/n3/pdf/v11n3a19.pdf

NATIONAL INDIAN FOUNDATION - FUNAI. **The Indians**. Available at: http://www.funai.gov.br/indios/conteudo.htm

LANGDON, E. J. **Illness as experience**: the construction of illness and its challenge for medical practice. 1995. Available at: http://www.cfh.ufsc.br/~nessi/A%20Doenca%20como%20Experienci a.htm

. **Health and Indigenous Peoples**: Challenges at the turn of the century. 1999. Available at: http://www.cfh.ufsc.br/~nessi/Margsav.htm

LAZZAROTTO, E. M.; BARATIERI, T.; (et.al.) **Existing diseases in the Kaingang and Guarani indigenous community**. 3rd National Seminar on the State and Social Policies in Brazil. UNIOESTE. 2007. Available at:

http://www.unioeste.br/prg/prolind/docs/doencas_existentes_comuni dade_indigena_kaingang_guarani.pdf

MORAES, J. C.; GARCIA, V. da G. L.; FONSECA, A. da S. Assistance provided in the adult intensive care unit: Clients' view. *Revista Nursing.* v.79, n.7, 2004. Available at: http://www.nursing.com.br/paper.php?p=214

MOURA, A. B. de M. **The national health care policy for indigenous peoples**. 2012. Available at: http://www.ufpe.br/remdipe/index.php?option=com_content&view=ar

ticle&id=395&Itemid=251

OLIVEIRA, P. S. de; NÓBREGA, M. M. L. da; SILVA, A. T. M. C. da; FERREIRA FILHA, M. de O. Therapeutic communication in nursing revealed in the testimonies of patients admitted to an Intensive Care Center. **Rev. Eletr. Enf**. 2005;7(1):54-63. Available   at:

http://www.fen.ufg.br/revista/revista7_1/original_05.htm

PELLON, L. H.; VARGAS, L. A. **Culture, interculturality and the health-disease process:** (dis)paths in health care for the Guarani Mbyà of   Aracruz,   Espirito   Santo.   2007.   Available   at: http://www.scielo.br/scielo.php?pid=S0103-73312010000400017&script=sci_arttext

ROLIM, K. M. C.; CARDOSO, M. V. L. M. L. The discourse and practice of care for newborns at risk: reflecting on humanized care. **Revista Latino-americana de Enfermagem** 2006, January-February; 14(1):85-92. Available at: http://www.scielo.br/pdf/rlae/v14n1/v14n1a12.pdf

SEGRE, M.; FERRAZ, F. C. **The concept of health**. 1997.

Available   at:
http://www.scielo.br/scielo.php?script=sci_arttext&pid=S0034-89101997000600016 Accessed on 10/06/2015.

SILVA, N. C. da; GONÇALVES, M. J. F.; LOPES NETO, D. **Enfermagem em saùde indigena**: aplicando as diretrizes curriculares; 2006. Available at:

http://www.scielo.br/scielo.php?script=sci_arttext&pid=S0034-71672003000400016

SIMOES, A. L. de A.; RODRIGUES, F. R.; TAVARES, D. M. dos S.; RODRIGUES, L. R. **Humanization in health**: focus on primary care. Texto Contexto Enferm, Florianópolis, 2007 Jul-Set; 16(3): 439-44. Available at:

http://www.rededepesquisaaps.org.br/UserFiles/File/Artigosinternaci
onais/artigonacional3.pdf

VIANNA, L. A. C. **Health-disease process**. 2012. Available at:
http://www.unasus.unifesp.br/biblioteca_virtual/esf/1/modulo_politico
_gestor/Unidade_6.pdf Accessed on: 16/06/2015.

VILA, V. da S. C.; ROSSI, L. A. The cultural meaning of humanized care
in the intensive care unit: "much talked about and little lived". **Rev.
Latino-americana de Enfermagem.** v. 10, n.° 02, p. 137   -   144,
2002. Available at:

http://www.scielo.br/pdf/rlae/v10n2/10506.pdf

WALDOL, V. R. **O cuidado na saùde**: as relações entre o eu, o outro e
o cosmos. Petropolis, RJ: Vozes, 2004.

10. CULTURAL ORAL HEALTH PREVENTION HABITS OF INDIGENOUS PEOPLES: A HISTORICAL ANALYSIS

RAFAEL DE PAULA MARCONDES, CLÓVIS LUCIANO GIACOMET

INTRODUCTION

Over the years, people's customs, way of life, technology, knowledge and education have changed a lot.

Cultural habits related to oral health prevention have also undergone many changes, and this is even more evident when it comes to indigenous health, as customs are even more different, as is the way of life and education.

This way of life, which is so different from that of the indigenous peoples, generates a great deal of curiosity both nationally and internationally. They can be said to be very acculturated to the culture of the white man in many villages, but also to have a rich culture and customs in others, from the way they eat, sanitize themselves, treat themselves, to herbal and mystical customs.

A country's development is linked to the health of its population. In dentistry, dental caries and periodontal diseases are prevalent diseases, as they are associated with social, economic, political and educational conditions.

Various barriers are encountered in dental care in indigenous villages, such as technological, linguistic, cultural, etc. However, the Indians' concerns about oral health range from appearance to its importance during chewing, since it is related to the ability to perform tasks within the community.

According to Arantes (2005):

Socio-economic variables end up defining greater or lesser access to preventive means, education and a less or more cariogenic diet. Cultural variables also play an important role in determining the disease, as they define dietary patterns, sugar consumption and the adoption of preventive methods. Behavioral variables are linked to individual behavior and include self-care and hygiene habits.

Indians have their own systems for interpreting, preventing and treating diseases, and although many advances have been made in the prevention and control of oral diseases, in indigenous oral health this evolution is primitive, since there is a lack of systematized information and there are no standards for recording dental activities.

According to research, there are around 4,200 indigenous communities distributed throughout Brazil, with approximately 225 ethnic groups, speaking more than 170 mother tongues.

The oral health of indigenous peoples is deteriorating, whether due to the consumption of industrialized foods or poor dental care, so that socio-economic, environmental and dietary changes are increasing the prevalence of caries in this population.

The aim of this research is to understand the habits of indigenous people in relation to oral health. As well as to identify the role of the dentist in oral health prevention; to describe the cultural habits of indigenous people in relation to oral health prevention; to analyze the history of indigenous oral health.

CULTURAL PREVENTION habits in oral HEALTH

In the view of the indigenous people, the dentist is seen as a "tooth puller", so that in the prevention of indigenous oral health it is essential, after understanding how they take care of themselves and without establishing rules, to act with availability and motivation, respecting the cultural aspects of the indigenous peoples, carrying out actions such as extraction and restoration, without the use of high or low rotation motors, only with manual cutting instruments, through atraumatic restorative treatment.

Among the methods used in oral health prevention today are the distribution of toothpastes and toothbrushes and the typical application of fluoride, whereas in the past, due to a more natural diet, the Indians kept their teeth healthy by chewing, since they consumed raw fruit and vegetables, which caused the teeth to self-clean, as they needed to be well-crushed, as well as eating plants.

So the ancestors prevented and fought toothache by applying ginger, which is good for toothache and sore throats, as well as herbal applications and natural solutions based on "medicinal" plants.

THE ROLE OF THE DENTIST IN ORAL HEALTH PREVENTION FOR INDIGENOUS PEOPLES

With the emergence of oral health promotion for the indigenous people, the need for new human resources also arose. According to Machado Jr. et.al. (2012):

When the inter-ethnic encounter - which takes place in the dentist/indigenous patient relationship in the village - is dissociated from this compression of sociocultural reality, dental work will be doomed to the job of removing dental elements, because it is still a stranger intervening in the village routine, teaching new hygiene habits and techniques that could directly interfere with the economy, social food taboos, local hygiene habits and concepts.

To this end, the role of the dentist in indigenous oral health prevention should emphasize self-care actions, valuing oral health and quality of life.

According to the author (2012):

The relationship between health professionals and patients, whatever their area of activity, goes far beyond the application of the technical knowledge they have acquired during their professional training.

He must promote interaction between the actions of "white" medicine and indigenous culture, providing curative and preventive care, organizing strategies for the implementation of an Oral Health Program.

Its role is to show the importance of preventing tooth decay, restorations and extractions, in a way that values traditional healing practices, helping to reduce the incidence of diseases such as tooth decay and improving their living conditions. According to Machado Jr. et.al. (2012):

The Oral Health Book presents, in addition to the themes of food and chewing from their myths and stories, the use of the plant called Wotch to clean teeth by the ancestors of the Ticuna people, and the use of a "dental floss" made from the leaves of the Tucumâ palm. Now, this initiative refers to indigenous autonomy - of the Ticuna, in the first instance - with regard to solving their own problems, in this case toothache and its complications, and this at any time, even in pre-Columbian and pre-Cabraline America.

Therefore, the dentist must have a humanistic, critical and reflective education, and must work at all levels of health care, with technical and scientific rigor, understanding the social, cultural and economic reality of his patient, since the indigenous population is concerned in terms of their oral health, using plants for dental impurities, Tucuma palm leaves as dental floss, medicinal plants in cases of pain, spells, charms, spiritual intervention, etc.

HISTORY OF INDIGENOUS PEOPLES' ORAL HEALTH

There are not many records on the issue of indigenous oral health, but it is known that the actions provided in the past were fragmented and lacked continuity, and were only curative in nature, rather than providing long-term treatment.

According to Arantes (2005) apud machado Jr. et.al. (2012):

"In general terms, there is a common trajectory in the oral health of indigenous peoples once they are in permanent contact with Western societies," but not the causality of tooth decay linked only to this contact, because, "Generally, these groups start from a situation of low to high prevalence of oral diseases, especially tooth decay [...] However, this pattern cannot be taken as a rule," he says....] However, this pattern cannot be taken as a rule," and from there he reports on what was seen in three indigenous groups in his research: the Xavante and the Enawenê-Nawê (from Mato Grosso), and the Guarani (from São Paulo). Curiously, the Enawenê-Nawê, who of the three peoples mentioned were the last to be contacted (1970s), and who maintain their traditional diet, had a higher rate of DMFT (decayed, lost or filled teeth) than the other two.

The first records of indigenous health care were reported by religious missions, and the Indian Protection Service (SPI), created in 1910 and which remained until 1967, was the first indigenous protection policy.

In 1956, the doctor and indigenist Noel Nutels institutionalized the SUSA, Serviço de Unidade Sanitària Aèrea, carrying out actions to control tuberculosis, vaccinations, communicable diseases and dental care (BERTANHA et.al., 2012).

With the creation of FUNAI, the National Indian Foundation, in 1967, by Decree Law No. 5371, it became responsible for their health care until 1999, when the National Health Foundation took over the care of indigenous peoples until 2010, the same year that the Subsystem was created through Law No. 9836/1999 or the Arouca Law, which encompassed the Special Indigenous Health Districts, providing basic care to the indigenous population, respecting their traditional systems and recognizing their social and cultural diversity. (BERTANHA et.al., 2012).

According to Cardoso de Oliveira (1972) apud

Machado Jr. et.al. (2012):

Based on his fieldwork among the Tücuna in Alto Solimoes-AM in the 1960s, he was the first to use the term "interethnic friction" to express the sociocultural phenomena following a tribal group's contact with national society, usually a confluent relationship.

While, according to Laraia (2004):

The fact that man sees the world through his culture means that he tends to consider his way of life as the most correct and natural. This tendency, called ethnocentrism, is responsible in its extreme cases for the occurrence of numerous social conflicts.

Regardless of ethnic and cultural differences, FUNAI's mission is to protect, promote and recover indigenous health in line with SUS policies and programs.

The indigenous population receives health care through the Indigenous Health Care Subsystem, which is integrated into the SUS in accordance with the guidelines of the National Policy for Health Care for Indigenous Peoples.

CULTURAL HABITS OF INDIGENOUS PEOPLE IN RELATION TO ORAL HEALTH PREVENTION

With changes in cultures and the political expansion of populations, we know that there have been huge changes in the actions and customs of the indigenous people, among which we must ask ourselves some questions, such as: what methods of oral health prevention were used in the past? How did their ancestors prevent and combat toothache? All this generates doubts and curiosities about the rich culture that preceded us.

According to Abreu (2005) apud Machado Jr. et.al. (2012):

Commenting on tooth decay in contemporary villages, he cites the research of dental surgeon Rui Arantes who, motivated by the desire to ascertain the existence of tooth decay among indigenous peoples, visited several Xavante villages in Mato Grosso in 1997, concluding that tooth decay had intensified in villages where the consumption of industrialized foods (oil, sugar, salt, soft drinks, etc.) from our society was more common.

There have been changes in the social, cultural, economic and intellectual structures of societies in general, including in the area of health. Many of the indigenous villages have undergone these changes and have adapted to the urban way of life, technological and acculturated to the white man.

Public policies aimed at indigenous people have changed housing, basic sanitation, education, social assistance, food and health, with dentistry standing out.

The more globalized world has introduced the influence of non-indigenous culture and customs into the daily life of the villages, thus changing oral health habits and care.

In the past, indigenous people's food was completely natural, that is, extracted from nature, such as fruits, roots, seeds, honey, hunting, fishing, herbs and agricultural production carried out by their own families and communities, growing beans, corn, manioc, rice and potatoes. Nowadays, the diet is more focused on industrialized food bought in shops in the cities, with access to refined sugar, sweets, soft drinks and other foods, which have such an influence on the development of tooth decay and dental problems.

On the other hand, there is also better access to fluoridated prevention products, high care methods, hygiene, access to the dentist, oral health education, thus obtaining practices that help and others that hinder oral health.

The Ministry of Health has a national policy guideline on indigenous oral health, which describes the functions and methods of individual and collective oral health promotion and protection, as well as recovery and rehabilitation in oral health (BRASIL, 2011).

Changes in diet (notably consumption of sugar and other industrialized products), related to socio-economic and environmental changes resulting from interaction with the surrounding national society, combined with the lack of preventive programs, are among the main causes of the deterioration in the oral health conditions of the Xavantes (ARANTES et AL, 2001).

As in other populations, indigenous peoples, in the case of tooth decay in particular, have a close relationship with cultural, behavioral and biological determinants (diet, exposure to fluoride, among others).

The number of cavities is attributed to the impact of changes in diet, associated with socio-economic and environmental changes and the lack of preventive programs.

As well as contributing to knowledge about the multi-causal age of tooth decay, research into indigenous oral health can generate relevant information for the planning and management of health services (ALVES FILHO et al, 2009). The intensity of the processes of socio-economic, cultural and environmental change, with wide-ranging impacts on health, is unquestionable.

Limited access to education and health services, conflicts over land and the absorption of indigenous people into regional markets have favored indigenous migration to Brazilian cities.

This entails a process of acculturation that leads to a food transition, as the population moves from subsistence activities based on hunting, fishing and gathering to the incorporation of industrialized foods, diverting their productive efforts to commercial crops in order to raise money to meet the needs created by the new socio-cultural habits.

In this context, it can be said that the accentuated and rapid cultural and environmental changes experienced by the diverse and different indigenous communities influence nutritional status and oral condition.

Furthermore, there is a need for intervention or monitoring through programs aimed at health care, basic sanitation, access to land and education, as well as longitudinal studies that can monitor the oral and nutritional conditions of these individuals and act to promote health for indigenous communities going through the process of dietary transition (MOURA et al, 2010).

CONCLUSION

This research into the cultural oral health prevention habits of indigenous peoples has shown that, in the past, the Indians carried out their dental treatments with the help of medicinal plants and herbs, as well as spells, charms, etc.

However, if we analyze the historical data on the oral health of indigenous peoples, there are few records of them. Oral diseases such as tooth decay only became part of the Indians' daily lives after the European intervention in this culture.

Faced with cultural differences, the role of the dentist is to seek to promote the prevention of oral health among indigenous peoples, through practices that are allied to their way of life and customs.

Further studies and research are still needed to gain a better understanding of the subject, as there are few articles and projects on the subject.

REFERENCES

ABREU, Cathia. **Toothache in the village?** 2005. Available at 216.70.94.79/toothache-in-the-village. Accessed on 12/05/2016.

ARANTES, Rui et al. **Oral health in the Xavànte indigenous population of Pimentel Barbosa, Mato Grosso, Brazil** Cad. Saùde Pùblica vol.17 no.2 Rio de Janeiro Mar./Apr. 2001

ARANTES, Rui. **Oral health of indigenous peoples in Brazil and the case of the Xavantes of Mato Grosso.** 2005. Available at www.arca.fiocruz.br/bistream/icict/

2/243.pdf. Accessed on 12/05/2016.

ALVES FILHO, Pedro et al. **Oral health of the Guarani Indians in the State of Rio de Janeiro, Brazil.** Cad. Saùde Pùblica vol.25 no.1 Rio de Janeiro Jan. 2009.

BERTANHA, Wânia de Fàtima Faraoni. et.al. **Oral health care in indigenous communities: evolution and challenges - a literature review.** 2012. PP.105-112. Available at

periódicos.ufpb.br/index.php/rbcs/article/viewfile/10116/7097.

Accessed on 13/05/2016.

ESCOBAR, Herton. **Book rescues Yanomami medicine and culture.** 2015. Available at ciência.estadao.com.br/noticias/geral,livro- resgata-medicina-e-cultura-ianomami,1744780. Accessed on 12/05/2016.

FGV, Getúlio Vargas Foundation. **Pioneering project presents the therapy of the Huni Kuin Indians.** 2014. Available at gvces.com.br/projeot-pioneiro-apresenta-a-terapeutica-dos-indios- huni-kuin?locale=EN.br. Accessed on 13/05/2016.

MACHADO JR, Eliseu Vieira. et.al. **Dentistry in the village: indigenous oral health from an anthropological perspective.** 2012. Available at http://revista.antropos.com.br/downloads/maio2012/Artigo7-OdontologianaAldeia.pdf. Accessed on 15/05/2016.

MOIMAZ, Suzely Adas Saliba. et.al. **Perception of oral health in an indigenous community in Brazil.** 2001. Available at www.unimep.br/phpg/editora/revistaspdf/revfol13_1art10pdf. Accessed on 15/05/2016.

NUNES, Selma A.C. **Avanços e desafios na implantaçâo da atençâo bàsica em saù.** 2003. Available at www.teses.usp.br/teses/disponiveis/25/25141/tde.../selmaaparecida chavesnunes.pdf Accessed on 15/05/2016.

MOURA, Patricia G. de et al. Indigenous population: a reflection on the influence of urban civilization on nutritional status and oral health. Rev. Nutr. vol.23 no.3 Campinas May/June 2010.

11. OBESITY IN INDIGENOUS POPULATIONS: AN APPROACH TO IMPROVING THE QUALITY OF LIFE.

Raisa Ottano Peixoto, Clóvis Luciano Giacomet

INTRODUCTION

According to ABESO - Associação Brasileira para o Estudo da Obesidade e da Sindrome Metabòlica (2014), obesity is considered by the WHO - World Health Organization - to be one of the world's biggest public health problems. By 2025, around 2.3 billion adults are expected to be overweight and more than 700 million obese. Among children, this figure would rise to 75 million if preventative actions are not developed as a matter of urgency.

In Brazil, according to a survey carried out by the Brazilian Institute of Geography and Statistics (IBGE) between 2008 and 2009, there has already been an increase in obesity rates, pointing out that, among adults, it has been estimated that around 50% of the population is overweight, i.e. in the overweight and obese range, and among children, the rate is around 15% (ABESO, 2014).

In addition, Mello (2004) states that obesity is a factor that has been growing significantly and causing various complications in childhood and adulthood and, according to Tenório, *et. al.* (2012), it stands out in society as a negative aspect, as there is a significant increase, gaining pandemic contours in both children and adults.

The Ministry of Health (2006) points out that obesity can be understood as "a multifactorial problem involving biological, historical, ecological, economic, social, cultural and political issues", given the changes that society has undergone over the years, which have also led to changes in people's habits, This has led to serious damage to health, such as sedentary lifestyles, especially among children, who live more in a virtual world than a real one, using their brains more than their bodies, eating more industrialized food than natural food, among other factors.

This whole scenario leads to the emergence of comorbidities that are of increasing concern to health professionals, who are seeing the number of people with obesity-related illnesses rise every day.

The situation is no different for indigenous people. Various studies and surveys show that the rates of obesity and related comorbidities are increasing significantly among the indigenous population.

The aim of this study is to investigate obesity rates among indigenous populations and the main comorbidities related to it.

OBESITY

According to the Ministry of Health (2006), obesity can be defined as "the degree of fat storage in the body associated with health risks, due to its relationship with various metabolic complications" and, according to Anjos (1992), "the basis of the disease is the undesirable process of positive energy balance, resulting in weight gain".

With regard to the etiology of obesity, ABESO (2009) states that it is complex and multifactorial, resulting from the interaction of genes, environment, lifestyles and emotional factors. The prevalence of obesity has been increasing significantly all over the world, making it a serious and worrying health problem, since it causes various health problems.

According to ABESO (2009):

There are three primary components of the neuroendocrine system involved in obesity: the afferent system, which involves leptin and other satiety and short-term appetite signals; the processing unit of the central nervous system; and the efferent system, a complex of appetite, satiety, autonomic and thermogenic effectors, which leads to energy storage.

As we can see, a variety of factors can lead to obesity and the strongest are environmental factors, with increased calorie intake and decreased levels of physical activity, promoted by the modern environment where *fast food* and excessive use of computers and electronic games, especially by children, are part of the routine of most people (ANJOS, 1992).

According to Coutinho (1998), the environment, cultural, economic and social factors, the intake of high-calorie foods, a reduction in physical activity, family structure and emotional factors are all contributing to the tendency towards obesity becoming more and more apparent at an earlier age.

CONTRIBUTING FACTORS TO OBESITY

As has already been pointed out, obesity has a multifactorial cause. Sigulem, *et.al.* (S/D) state that family history is very important in determining the occurrence of obesity and other eating disorders. According to the authors, a child with obese parents has an 80% chance of presenting the same profile, and this risk drops by half if only one of the parents is obese. If neither parent is obese, the child has a 7% risk of becoming obese. However, the research reported by Sigulem, *et.al.* (S/D) does not define exactly to what extent genetic inheritance influences obesity and how much is due to the family environment in which the child lives.

In addition to the genetic factor, there are also environmental factors such as diet and a sedentary lifestyle.

With regard to emotional factors, Sigulem (S/D) states that "eating behavior is a very complex phenomenon which involves cognitive aspects, social and emotional development", since obese people seem to respond more to external stimuli such as the type and quality of food than to internal stimuli such as hunger and satiety in relation to appetite. Campos, *et.al.* (1985) also hypothesized that some children experience greater oral gratification than other satisfactions, which leads to greater food consumption, in this case due to the inheritance of psychic structures, thus configuring an emotional and psychological factor.

FOOD

Adequate nutrition from childhood onwards is essential not only for the child's growth and development, but also for our survival, as it is at this stage that good eating habits are established, which must be maintained into adolescence (LAMOUNIER; ABRANTES, 2003).

At this stage, eating habits are greatly influenced by advertising and fads that encourage the consumption of more energy-dense foods, associated with little physical activity, which can contribute to the development of obesity, a problem that is increasing among young people (OLIVEIRA; VEIGA, 2005).

Garcia, Gambardella and Frutuoso (2003) report, based on a survey of adolescents, that their diet is characterized by foods with inadequate nutritional value, i.e. those high in saturated fat and cholesterol, as well as a large amount of salt and sugar. Excessive consumption of these foods can lead to an increase in body fat and, as a result, overweight and obesity.

When it comes to food consumption, some authors have observed that adolescents have an inadequate dietary practice, generally with an intake of total and saturated fat above the recommended level, and a deficient intake of certain vitamins and minerals (SANTOS, 2003).

During the growth phase, children and adolescents often need to eat more frequently and in larger quantities. However, when growth slows down, they need to be more careful, as excessive eating habits during this phase of life can contribute to the appearance of overweight and obesity, among other chronic degenerative diseases (SANTOS, 2003).

INFLUENCE OF POOR DIET

The increase in obesity is the result of early and incorrect weaning, due to dietary errors in the first years of life, where parents abandon breastfeeding and switch to foods with large amounts of carbohydrates, which are more than children need for their growth and development (FREITAS; COELHO; RIBEIRO, 2009).

The lack of care taken with children's diets can be seen from their earliest years, showing that this lack may be directly affecting obesity.

In addition, quick and tasty snacks that attract attention are becoming more and more common in children's lives, making eating these nutrient-poor foods a routine and thus contributing to overweight.

Fast food and the excessive consumption of industrialized products are one of the factors contributing to the increase in obesity, with an 82% increase in the Brazilian population. In these meals, the high caloric value of fats and sugars increases the total caloric density of the meals (SILVEIRA; ABREU, 2006).

In addition, these factors contribute to main meals being left out, as they reduce appetite and make children lose interest in the main foods that are ideal for healthy growth.

The main dietary deviations include: insufficient consumption of fruit, vegetables, legumes (especially beans), skipping meals, especially breakfast, reducing milk consumption, switching to milk drinks with a lower calcium concentration, increasing consumption of ready-made and frozen products, as well as soft drinks (RINALDI et al., 2008).

Parents play a fundamental role in children's diets, as they should be guiding them and setting rules for their diet, as well as advising them on the benefits and harms that inadequate nutrition can cause in the coming years of their lives.

The family is responsible for the way children eat through social learning, with parents being the main nutritional educators. The social context plays a major role in the learning process, mainly through the way parents teach children to eat or to learn to eat specific foods. The way in which they are taught can provide both adequate and inadequate stimuli in defining children's food preferences (MOURA, 2010).

OBESITY IN INDIGENOUS POPULATIONS

According to Souza and Alves (2013), the indigenous population has grown by around 205% in the last twenty years, totaling approximately nine hundred thousand people who are distributed throughout the country in different proportions according to the regions, with around 40% of this population currently living in urban areas, according to data from the last Census carried out by the IBGE in 2010.

Lourenço (2006) carried out a study on the nutritional status in relation to socio-economic aspects of indigenous adults in an indigenous population in Rondônia and warned that the socio-cultural and economic transformation caused by the growing contact between indigenous populations and non-indigenous society has altered their habits, especially with regard to food, causing changes in their health.

Pyl (2014) reports in his article that a study carried out by endocrinologist João Paulo Botelho Vieira Filho found that the gradual abandonment of the indigenous people's traditional diet, as well as a reduction in the physical effort of hunting, fishing and traditional agriculture, in addition to the introduction of industrialized foods such as refined sugar and rice (supplied by the Federal Government itself).

The doctor has been studying the causes of diabetes, overweight and obesity since the 1970s among the Xavante Indians of Mato Grosso and the Xikrin, Surui and Gavião of Pará. He explains that among the Xavante, after the Rice Project, promoted by FUNAI in 1981, the Indians began to consume the cereal at every meal, even adding sugar in the morning, as well as progressively abandoning the bean fields, carà, pumpkin, peanuts, manioc and other products collected in the forests, such as inajâ coconut, cerrado roots, grasshoppers and babaçu larvae, important sources of protein that are no longer part of the indigenous diet.

Viera Filho says that type 2 diabetes is an epidemic among the indigenous people of Brazil and the cause is a change in eating habits. He explains that there is also a genetic factor: the ABCA1 gene, which is only present in natives of the Americas and is linked to the accumulation of energy and fat to protect the body during periods of drought and hunger. With an excessive intake of sugar and fat, the body goes out of control and diabetes occurs.

In 2015, Vieira Filho published an article in a North American magazine, in which he pointed out that in a population of 948 Xavante Indians from Mato Grosso, 28.2% were found to have diabetes, of which 40.6% were women and 18.4% men, while 17.5% were diagnosed with hypertension and half were considered obese.

In view of this scenario, Souza and Alves (2013) warn that the indigenous population is vulnerable to food and nutritional problems, ranging from obesity to malnutrition.

According to anthropologist Paulo Santilli, the fact that has driven the increase in the consumption of industrialized food in recent years has been the creation of various social assistance programs by the Federal Government, favoring access to industrialized food and household appliances, especially for the elderly and children, to the detriment of cultivation, fishing and hunting to make a living. These transformations in the way of life do not mean that the Indians are losing their identity, but rather that it is possible to adapt to the new conditions and seek a better quality of life through these resources (DIAS; SANTILLI, 2014).

Menezes and Schauren (2015) report on a study carried out in four Terena villages in Mato Grosso do Sul in which they assessed the population's eating habits and found that there had been a significant increase in the consumption of industrialized products and sugar, salt, soybean oil, powdered milk, tomato extract, powdered soft drinks, tea, soft drinks, sweets, French bread and sausages, some of which make up the food basket provided by the state government.

Other products consumed by indigenous people such as soft drinks, snacks, sweets and alcoholic beverages, which are prohibited by indigenous communities, are used by those who have their own resources such as pensions or salaries from some kind of work or even from selling handicraft products and are part of the dietary routine of the indigenous people surveyed (MENEZES; SHAUREN, 2015).

A study carried out by Santos, *et.al.* (2012) also found a high consumption of industrialized products and beef, which had not previously been part of the indigenous diet. Although the staple diet is still beans, rice and corn, many other products such as soluble coffee, macaroni and cookies are introduced in ever greater quantities and the author also warns of the high consumption of alcoholic drinks, products which increase the rates of type 2 diabetes and hypertension among the indigenous population.

CONSEQUENCES OF OBESITY IN INDIGENOUS POPULATIONS

As mentioned above, the natives of the Americas have the ABCA1 gene, which is linked to the accumulation of energy and fat to protect the body during periods of drought and hunger. This factor, coupled with the change in eating habits caused by the ever-increasing process of acculturation of indigenous people through coexistence with non-indigenous societies, ends up causing a series of diseases that were not part of the lives of indigenous populations, such as hypertension and type 2 diabetes.

With regard to hypertension in the Brazilian indigenous population, Bloch, et.al. (1993) states that during the early 1990s, published studies revealed that these specific populations had average systemic and diastolic blood pressures below those of the Brazilian population. However, a more recent study found higher averages of systemic blood pressure in these specific communities (BLOCH, *et al.*, 1993).

Lunardi, Santos and Coimbra Jr. (2007) also highlight cases of hypertension in the Xavante ethnic group in Mato Grosso, bringing up the debate about changes in their lifestyle habits. A study conducted with indigenous populations in Rio de Janeiro points out that one of the most obvious causes of the identification of cases of hypertension is the change in lifestyle attributed to a process of civilization that the Indians have been undergoing (CARDOSO; MATTOS; KOIFMAN, 2001).

In relation to type 2 diabetes mellitus, Vieira Filho (1992), in the 1990s, already observed a prevalence of obesity among the Xavante of Sangradouro and São Marcos of 50.8%, diabetes of 28.2% (18.4% in men and 40.6% in women), glucose intolerance of 32.3% (29.7% in men and 34.4% in women) and hypertension of 17.5% among 948 Indians aged between 15 and 99.

According to this author, Indians have genetics favorable to obesity, metabolic syndrome, diabetes mellitus with more serious complications due to the ABCA1 gene, already mentioned above and this, combined with changes in eating habits, contributes to the situation getting worse and worse.

CONCLUSION

It has been observed that obesity has become a public health problem in both developed and developing countries. This can be attributed to changes in people's eating habits, with a large consumption of industrialized products containing excess fat and sugar, as well as other factors, such as the influence of the media, for example.

Along with obesity, comorbidities such as hypertension and diabetes are growing alarmingly and are responsible for a large percentage of mortality due to factors resulting from them.

In relation to indigenous populations, the focus of this study, it was observed through the studies carried out that the situation is no different, as indigenous people also have high rates of obesity and, associated with it, hypertension and diabetes as the main resulting diseases.

This increase in obesity among indigenous people is mainly due to the process of acculturation that these populations have undergone since the colonization of the country, as more and more primitive habits are abandoned in favor of non-indigenous practices, such as the consumption of large-scale industrialized foods, alcoholic beverages and the gradual abandonment of the production of natural foods for consumption.

Studies on the subject are sparse. Few bibliographical references were found on diabetes, and even then they were very old, which makes it impossible to get a real sense of the problem, demonstrating that there is no real interest on the part of the competent bodies in controlling the problem. On the contrary, with the supply of food baskets by the state and federal governments, which contain a large number of industrialized foods, the tendency is for the situation to get even worse.

It is true that public health care policies are trying to minimize the problem, but coordinated and joint action is needed so that priorities can be established and the population can be served in a way that is closer to the dietary reeducation they had before contact with non-indigenous civilizations.

We therefore conclude that the initial objective of the study was achieved and that it will greatly contribute to the professional practice of the researcher who works in the area of indigenous health.

REFERENCES

ANJOS, Luiz A. **indice de massa corporal (massa corporal estatura-2) como indicador do estado nutricional de adultos**: revisâo da literatura. Revista de Saùde Pùblica, Sâo Paulo, v. 26, n. 6, p. 431-436, 1992.

BRAZILIAN ASSOCIATION FOR THE STUDY OF OBESITY AND METABOLIC SYNDROME. **Map of obesity**. 2014. Available at:
http://www.abeso.org.br/atitude-saudavel/mapa-obesidade
Accessed on 25/08/2015.

BRAZILIAN ASSOCIATION FOR THE STUDY OF OBESITY AND METABOLIC SYNDROME. **Brazilian obesity guidelines 2009/2010.** 3.ed. - Itapevi, SP: AC Farmacêutica, 2009.

BLOCH, Katia V.; *et.al.* Blood pressure, capillary glycemia and anthropometric measurements in a Yanomami population. **Cadernos de Saùblica,** 9:428-438, 1993. Available at:
http://www.scielo.br/scielo.php?script=sci arttext&pid=S0102-311X1993000400003 Accessed on 12/05/2016.

BRAZIL. Ministry of Health. Department of Primary Care. **Obesity**. Brasilia: Ministry of Health, 2006. Available at:
http://189.28.128.100/dab/docs/publicacoes/cadernos ab/abcad12.p df
Accessed on 12/05/2016.

CAMPOS, Fernando Antonio C.A.; CAMPOS, Flavio R.A.; CUNHA JR, Hilton P. da; ALBUQUERQUE, João de. Etiology of obesity in infants. **Jornal de Pediatria** 58 (4) -, 1985. Available at: http://www.ufscar.br/~efe/pdf/2a/colloca.pdf Accessed on 03/05/2016.

CARDOSO, Andrey M.; MATTOS, Inês E.; KOIFMAN, Rosalina J. Prevalência de fatores de risco para doenças cardiovasculares na PopulaQão Guarani-Mbyà do Estado do Rio de Janeiro. **Cadernos de Saùde Pùblica,** 17:345-354, 2001. Available at: http://www.scielosp.org/pdf/csp/v17n2/4179.pdf Accessed at 21/05/2016.

COUTINHO, Walmir. **Etiology of obesity**. 1998. Available at: http://www.abeso.org.br/uploads/downloads/18/552fea46a6bb6.pdf Accessed on 02/05/2016.

DIAS, Laercio; SANTILLI, Paulo. **Brazilian Indians develop "Urban" diseases after lifestyle changes**. UNESP. Araraquara, Brazil, 2014. Available at: http://saudeamanha.fiocruz.br/%C3%ADndios-brasileiros-develop-urban-diseases-after-change-in-lifestyle Accessed on 12/05/2016.

FREITAS, Andréa Silva de Souza; COELHO, Simone Cortêz; RIBEIRO, Ricardo Laino. Childhood obesity: Influence of inadequate eating habits. **Revista Saùde & Ambiente** 2009, v.4, n.2, pp. 09-14. Available at: http://publicacoes.unigranrio.br/index.php/sare/article/view/613/598 Accessed on 17/04/2016.

GARCIA, Christina Barbosa; GAMBARDELLA, Ana Maria Dianezi; FRUTUOSO, Maria Fernanda Petrole. Nutritional status and food consumption of adolescents at a youth center in the city of Sao Paulo. **Rev. Nutr., Campinas,** 16(1):41-50, jan./mar., 2003. Available at:

http://www.scielo.br/pdf/rn/v16n1/a04v16n1 Accessed on 12/04/2016.

LAKATOS, Eva Maria; MARCONI, Mariana de Andrade. **Metodologia do trabalho cientifico: procedimentos bàsicos, pesquisa bibliogràfica, projeto e relatório publicaçôes e trabalhos cientificos.** 2 ed. Sao Paulo: Atlas, 1987.

LAMOUNIER, Joel Alves; ABRANTES, Marcelo Militao. Prevalence of obesity and overweight in adolescence in Brazil. **Rev Med**

Minas Gerais 2003; 13(4):275-84. Available at:

https://www.nescon.medicina.ufmg.br/biblioteca/imagem/1809.pdf Accessed on 13/05/2016.

LOURENÇO, A. E. P. **Evaluation of the nutritional status in relation to socio-economic aspects of Surui indigenous adults, Rondônla, Brazil.** 2006. 77f. Master's degree dissertation. ENSP/ FIOCRUZ, Rio de Janeiro, 2006. Available at: http://arca.icict.fiocruz.br/handle/icict/5068 Accessed on 01/04/2016.

LUNARDI, Rosaline; SANTOS, Ricardo Ventura; COIMBRA JUNIOR, Carlos E.A. Morbidade hospitalar de indìgenas Xavante, Mato Grosso, Brasil (2000-2002). **Rev. bras. epidemiol.** vol.10 no.4 Sâo Paulo Dec. 2007. Available at at:

http://www.scielo.br/scielo.php?script=sci arttext&pid=S1415-790X2007000400002 Accessed on 21/05/2016.

MELLO, Elza D.; LUFT, Vician; MEYER, Flavia. Childhood ohesity: how can we be effective? Jornal de Pediatria - Vol. 80, N°3, 2004. Available at: http://www.scielo.br/pdf/jped/v80n3/v80n3a04 Accessed on 29/04/2016.

MOURA, Neila Camargo de. Influence of the media on the eating behavior of children and adolescents. **Segurança Alimentar e Nutricional**, Campinas, 17(1): 113-122, 2010. Available at:

http://www.unicamp.br/nepa/publicacoes/san/2010/XVII 1/docs/influ encia-da-midia-no-comportamento-alimentar-de-criancas-e- adolescentes.pdf Accessed on 03/05/2016.

OLIVEIRA, Celina Szuchmacher; VEIGA, Glória Valéria da. Nutritional status and sexual maturation of adolescents from a public school and a private school in the municipality of Rio de Janeiro. **Rev Nutr. Campinas**. Vol. 18. No. 2. 2005. Available at: http://www.scielo.br/pdf/rn/v18n2/24374.pdf Accessed on 28/04/2016.

OLIVEIRA, Geraldo Ferreira de. Prevalence of cardiometabolic risk factors in an indigenous community in central Brazil: a population-based cross-sectional study. 2014. 94 f., il. Thesis (Doctorate in Health Sciences) -University of Brasilia, Brasilia, 2014.

PYL, Bianca. **Territory and food sovereignty**: challenges for Indians in São Paulo. Pro-Indian Commission. 2014. Available at: http://www.cpisp.org.br/indios/upload/editor/files/MateriaSoberaniaAl imentarProIndio.pdf Accessed on 05/04/2016.

RINALDI, Ana Elisa M. *et.al.* Contributions of dietary practices and physical inactivity to childhood overweight. **Rev Paul Pediatr** 2008;26(3):271-7. Available at at: http://www.scielo.br/pdf/rpp/v26n3/12.pdf Accessed on 20/04/2016.

SANTOS, Andréia Mendes dos. The overweight family with childhood obesity. **Revista Virtual Textos & Contextos**, n° 2, dec. 2003. Available at at: http://revistaseletronicas.pucrs.br/ojs/index.php/fass/article/viewFile/ 964/744 Accessed on 04/05/2016.

SANTOS, Kenedy Maia dos. *et al.* Degree of physical activity and metabolic syndrome: a cross-sectional study with Khisêdsê Indians from the Xingu Park, Brazil. **Caderno de Saùblica**. Rio de Janeiro, v. 12, n. 3,

p. 153-160, 2012.

SIGULEM, Dirce Maria; *et.al*. Obesity in childhood and adolescence. **Compacta Nutriçâo**. UNESP-EPM. (S/D). São Paulo.

SILVEIRA, Samara; ABREU, Solange Malentachi. Factors contributing to childhood obesity. **Rev Enferm UNISA** 2006; 7: 59-62   .

Available at   at:

http://www.unisa.br/graduacao/biologicas/enfer/revista/arquivos/200   6-11.pdf Accessed on 01/05/2016.

SOUZA, Karina Lavinia P. do Carmo Régis de; ALVES, Crésio de Aragâo Dantas. Nutritional diagnosis of indigenous children and adults attended by the public health network in Brazil: an exploratory study. **Rev. Ciênc. Méd. Biol.**, Salvador, v.12, especial, p.433440, dez.2013.   Available at   at:

http://www.portalseer.ufba.br/index.php/cmbio/article/view/9187 Accessed on 12/04/2016.

TENÓRIO, Luis Henrique S.; *et.al*. Obesity and pulmonary function tests in children and adolescents: a systematic review. **Rev Paul Pediatr** 2012;30(3):423-30.   Available   at: http://www.scielo.br/pdf/rpp/v30n3/18.pdf Accessed on 12/04/2016.

VIEIRA FILHO, Joâo Paulo Botelho. Diabetes mellitus and the fasting glucose levels of the Caripuna and Palikur Indians. **Rev Ass Med Brasil**.   23(5):175-178,   1992. Available at:

http://www.scielo.br/scielo.php?script=sci   nlinks&ref=000134&pid=S 0102-311X200100020000600034&lng=en Accessed on 04/06/2016.

12. HEALTH CARE AT INDIGENOUS WOMEN DURING PREGNANCY

Simone Aparecida da Silva, Clóvis Luciano Giacomet

INTRODUCTION

Women have historically come from a background of exclusion in all areas, being seen as a supporting figure in family life, with the main role being reproduction, childbearing and caring for the home and family, with virtually no social rights (to study, work, etc.).

In Brazil, women were only allowed to attend schools in 1827, and even then, only elementary schools, since they were not allowed to attend higher education institutions, and were only authorized to do so in 1879, but those who dared to do so were severely criticized by society, They were even socially excluded, as it was considered at the time that a woman's place was in the home, learning "domestic chores" from their mothers, who had learned them from their grandmothers, perpetuating a culture of excluding women from other areas of social life (HAHNER, 2003).

There are various concepts of women's health in the literature. There are narrower concepts that deal only with aspects of the biology and anatomy of the female body, and broader ones that interact with dimensions of human rights and citizenship issues. In the narrower conceptions, women's bodies are seen only in terms of their reproductive function and motherhood becomes their main attribute. Women's health is limited to maternal health or the absence of illness associated with the process of biological reproduction. In this case, sexual rights and gender issues are excluded (COELHO, 2003).

As far as indigenous women's health is concerned, it is covered in a non-specific way in the National Policy for Comprehensive Care for Women's

Health, in a broad way, disregarding the specifics of the traditional indigenous health care system.

As far as specific care for indigenous pregnant women is concerned, there is a scarcity of scientific work on the subject, which sparked an interest in deepening our knowledge by searching the existing literature for support.

The aim of this study is to investigate how care for indigenous pregnant women is provided in Brazil, using bibliographic research as a methodology, searching for articles on *sites* such as Scielo, the Virtual Health Library (BVS), as well as theses and dissertations for the necessary references.

CONTEXTUALIZING INDIGENOUS HEALTH ACTIONS

Around 1910, health care for indigenous peoples was the responsibility of the Indian Protection Service (SPI). In this sense, indigenous health care began to receive greater assistance from the state, and the recovery of the health of the 31 indigenous groups identified in Brazil in the face of the epidemics that emerged at that time was one of the state's first actions (BRASIL, 2002).

With the extinction of the Indian Protection Service in 1967, the National Indian Foundation (FUNAI) was created and established sectors to deal with the health problems of the indigenous populations. According to Bernardes (2011), indigenous health care began to be provided by a mobile health team. This team was responsible for attending to the indigenous communities in its area of operation, providing medical assistance, administering vaccines and supervising local health work.

Health posts were also set up in indigenous areas to meet the primary health needs of the communities (BRASIL, 2002). In the 1990s, indigenous health ceased to be taken care of by FUNAI and became the responsibility of the Ministry of Health through the National Health Foundation (FUNASA), which has Special Indigenous Health Districts (DSEI), which are local health units, guaranteeing indigenous peoples full access to health, taking into account ethnic and cultural specificities, through this subsystem integrated into the Unified Health System (BERNARDES, 2011).

In August 2010, the Special Secretariat for Indigenous Health (SESAI) was created. This creation of a specific secretariat for Indigenous Health resulted in the transfer of actions to the Ministry of Health. According to Brasil (2009), this Secretariat is responsible for coordinating and executing the management process of the Indigenous Health Care Subsystem throughout the national territory, with the protection, promotion and recovery of the health of indigenous peoples as its responsibility, in line with the public policies and programs established by the Unified Health System (SUS).

In relation to women's health, it is integrated into the National Policy for Women's Health Care

THE NATIONAL POLICY FOR COMPREHENSIVE WOMEN'S HEALTH CARE

In Brazil, women's health was incorporated into national health policies in the first decades of the 20th century, and during this period it was limited to the demands of pregnancy and childbirth. The maternal and child programs drawn up in the 1930s, 1950s and 1970s reflected a restricted view of women, based on their biological specificity and their social role as mothers and housewives, responsible for raising, educating and caring for the health of their children and other family members (BRASIL, 2004).

According to Costa (1999), there are analyses that show that these programs advocated maternal and child actions as a strategy to protect groups at risk and in situations of greater vulnerability, such as children and pregnant women. Another characteristic of these programs was their verticality and lack of integration with other programs and actions proposed by the federal government. The targets were set by the central level, without any assessment of the health needs of the local populations. One of the results of this practice is the fragmentation of care and the low impact on women's health indicators.

With greater demands from society, driven by the feminist movement that arrived in Brazil in 1984, the Ministry of Health drew up the Program for Comprehensive Assistance to Women's Health (PAISM), marking, above all, a conceptual break with the guiding principles of women's health policy and the criteria for choosing priorities in this field (BRASIL, 1984).

The PAISM incorporated as its principles and guidelines the proposals of decentralization, hierarchization and regionalization of services, as well as the integrality and equity of care, at a time when the conceptual system that would form the basis for the formulation of the Unified Health System (SUS) was being conceived within the Health Movement.

This program included educational, preventive, diagnostic, treatment and recovery actions, including care for women in gynecological clinics, prenatal care, childbirth and puerperium, climacteric care, family planning, STDs, cervical and breast cancer, as well as other needs identified based on the population profile of women (BRASIL, 1984).

This program constituted women's health care until 2004, when the National Policy for Comprehensive Women's Health Care - PNAISM - was launched by the Ministry of Health, in view of the need to recognize the need for guidelines for public policies on women's health (BRASIL, 2004).

According to the Ministry of Health, the main objectives of the National Policy for Comprehensive Women's Health Care are: - To promote the improvement of the living conditions and health of Brazilian women, through the guarantee of legally constituted rights and the expansion of access to the means and services of health promotion, prevention, assistance and recovery throughout the Brazilian territory.

- To contribute to the reduction of female morbidity and mortality in Brazil, especially from preventable causes, in all life cycles and in the various population groups, without discrimination of any kind.

- To expand, qualify and humanize comprehensive care for women's health in the Unified Health System.

With regard to its actions, the PNAISM points to humanized care as a priority, with the main focus on the following situations:

-     Maternal mortality, with subdivisions covering: precarious obstetric care; abortion in precarious conditions; precarious contraceptive care; STD/HIV/AIDS;

-     Domestic and sexual violence;

-     The health of adolescent women;

-     Women's health in the climacteric/menopause;

-     Mental health and gender;

-     Chronic degenerative diseases and gynecological cancer;

-     Black women's health;

-     Indigenous women's health;

-     Lesbian women's health;

-     Health of women living and working in rural areas;

-     The health of women in prison.

Within the scope of PNAISM, some aspects considered essential in the implementation of actions should also be highlighted: the humanization of care, in the sense of learning to share knowledge and recognize rights. Good quality, humanized care implies establishing relationships between individuals who are similar, even though they may be very different according to their social, racial, ethnic, cultural and gender conditions, and the need to consider local specificities when implementing the policy (BRASIL, 2004).

INDIGENOUS WOMEN'S HEALTH

As has already been pointed out, indigenous women's health is linked to the PNAISM, but without any specifics, and the guidelines themselves contain the following statement: Attention to indigenous women's health is still precarious, and actions such as prenatal care, cervical cancer prevention, STD/HIV/AIDS prevention, among others, have not been guaranteed. There is still insufficient epidemiological data available to assess the health problems of the population of indigenous women and adolescents. It is essential to develop health policies aimed at these women, in the context of the ethno-development of indigenous societies and comprehensive care, involving indigenous communities in defining and monitoring them (BRASIL, 2004).

HEALTH CARE FOR INDIGENOUS WOMEN DURING PREGNANCY

As there is no specific reference in the National Policy for Comprehensive Women's Health Care, other studies were used in order to gather information for this research.

Moliterno, *et.al.* (2013), carried out a study in the Indigenous Land of Faxinal de Catanduva-PR, which has around 600 residents, distributed in approximately 120 families. It is located in the municipality of Càndido de

Abreu, in the central-southern region of Paranà and they found that there is a Basic Health Unit in the village, where pregnant women receive prenatal care provided by doctors and nurses.

When the time comes to give birth, pregnant women are taken to the nearest hospital. However, some of the women in the village still prefer the "traditional" way of giving birth, as they learned from their mothers and grandmothers (MOLITERNO, *et.al.*, 2013).

They also show that pregnant women prepare from the beginning of the pregnancy, reporting that they resort to rituals of the tribe, using herbs to inhibit the growth of the fetus and make it better positioned, thus facilitating childbirth, given that the baby doesn't grow much. They also reduce the amount of food they eat, but take herbal remedies to make the baby "strong". The authors hypothesize that the above factors could be the cause of the Kaingang's short stature, which is lower than the national average for non-Indians (MOLITERNO, *et.al.*, 2013).

Another factor observed by the researchers was the naturalness with which the indigenous women treat childbirth at home and squatting, usually alone, closed up in the house or, when it's the first child, the mother or a midwife accompanies to "teach" how it's done, and in other deliveries, the pregnant woman has to manage on her own (MOLITERNO, *et.al.*, 2013).

After childbirth, the umbilical cord and placenta are buried along with the bush remedies that were used before the birth to ease the pain. The authors explain that this is due to the indigenous people's strong relationship with the land, believing that their roots are there and that their bodies should be buried in the same place.

This practice, however, was observed among the older indigenous women, while most of the younger ones opted for hospital care, giving birth assisted by obstetricians and a health team, demonstrating that the process of acculturation has influenced indigenous women's perceptions of pregnancy and childbirth.

In the reports from pregnant women who have their babies in a hospital environment, the complaints are about the form of care, which does not take into account the cultural values of indigenous women. Hospital care restricts the parturient woman to a horizontal position, highlighting the clash between indigenous culture and the obstetric routine in maternity hospitals. It was observed that Kaingang women are very uncomfortable with the position to which they are subjected for the birth of their children in an institution, since remaining in dorsal decubitus is not in line with their conceptions of how to give birth, contrary to the physiology of childbirth, in which the different perspectives endowed with cultural values should be respected whenever possible (MOLITERNO, et.al., 2013).

It is clear that there is no differentiated treatment that takes into account the cultural differences and perceptions of indigenous pregnant women at the time of childbirth. The testimonies show how irrelevant the choices and opinions of the women are to the professionals, highlighting the supremacy of the technical and interventionist training of the medical professional who disregards the preparation of the indigenous woman and her choice for natural childbirth. It is also clear that these women have lost the possibility of actively participating in their births, since the professionals are the only ones responsible for deciding on the procedures to be implemented during hospitalization (MOLITERNO, et.al., 2013).

The care received by indigenous pregnant women when they opt for hospital delivery was reported by the authors as the biggest factor in their rejection of hospital medical care at the time of delivery, highlighting the importance and need for health professionals to respect the various aspects of women, seeing them as an integral being, endowed with their own social and cultural principles (MOLITERNO, *et.al.*, 2013).

In the research by Menezes (2012), carried out in a Guarani-mbyà village in the northwest of the state of São Paulo, it was also observed that the majority of births take place in a hospital environment, in the case of younger mothers, while older mothers still prefer the traditional way of giving birth at home.

Pregnant women who opted for a hospital birth reported that it was easier because they didn't feel as much pain and the birth was quicker.

What is striking in the report by Menezes (2012) is the fact that pregnant women ask to take the placenta home and the hospital refuses. As Moliterno, et.al. (2013) mentioned, the burial of the placenta and part of the umbilical cord is part of indigenous beliefs and customs, but this is not taken into account, demonstrating a lack of appreciation for indigenous culture and often leading pregnant women to choose to give birth at home.

As a positive experience in the care of indigenous pregnant women, a reference was found at the Nossa Senhora de Nazareth Maternal and Child Hospital (HMINSN), in Boa Vista, Roraima, which welcomes indigenous pregnant women with specialized care aimed at valuing the patient's culture (BRASIL, 2016).

However, this is the only maternity hospital in the whole country that provides this type of care. The maternity hospital has had an Indigenous Coordination for over sixteen years and is responsible for coordinating care so that indigenous pregnant women can practice their customs without risking themselves, their babies or other patients.

Within the Indigenous Coordination there are indigenous language interpreters at the disposal of the health professionals, facilitating the link between the pregnant women and them, providing opportunities to develop actions that value indigenous culture.

The care team includes a nursing technician, who is the indigenous coordinator and has been doing so for over fourteen years. She speaks four indigenous mother tongues and also acts as an interpreter. In addition to her, four other trained professionals provide care.

In this way, indigenous pregnant women have their customs respected and valued, so that the moment of birth, even in a hospital environment, is humanized and as close as possible to a home birth.

CONCLUSION

At the end of this research work, we highlight the scarcity of scientific papers on the subject, making it difficult to provide a theoretical basis for the research and demonstrating a gap to be filled in terms of scientific research exploring the subject.

It was found that women have a historically constructed history of exclusion, which has only been transformed after many movements in favor of emancipation and the valorization of gender. However, many actions in the form of public policies are still needed for women to be conceived as subjects with full rights.

With regard to women's health, it was found that until 2004, there were no specific actions in the area of care and it was only after the implementation of the National Policy for Comprehensive Care for Women's Health that the scenario began to show changes in the care given to women's health, with effective and concrete actions.

In relation to indigenous women's health, no reference was found to differentiated care in this policy, and the Ministry of Health itself recognizes that indigenous women's health care is precarious, requiring an urgent rethink of the issue.

With regard to care for indigenous pregnant women, it can be concluded that it is provided in Basic Health Units, but without any differentiation in the model of care, and therefore does not take into account the cultural specificities, beliefs and values of indigenous peoples, which, in most cases, keeps pregnant women away from care.

It was interesting to see that the process of acculturation that indigenous societies are going through due to coexistence with non-indigenous societies and the change in habits and customs, has also led to the perception of younger indigenous pregnant women, who prefer hospital births, even when they have to adapt to the extremely technical model of care, which does not respect indigenous beliefs, such as the refusal to take the placenta to be buried.

We found only one maternity hospital in the whole country where indigenous pregnant women have the opportunity to give birth in hospital, in a way that respects and values the traditions of their ethnic group, which should happen in all states with indigenous populations.

Finally, the bibliographical research has given rise to the need and desire, as a health professional working in indigenous communities, to delve deeper into the subject by carrying out field research, where the perceptions of indigenous pregnant women about conception, pregnancy and childbirth can be closely observed and analyzed, so that a parallel can be drawn with the studies found and perhaps contribute to scientific production on the subject.

REFERENCES

BERNARDES, Anita Guazzelli. Indigenous health and public policies: alterity and the state of exception. **Interface - Comunicação, Saùde e Educaçâo**, v. 15, n. 36, p. 153-64, jan./mar. 2011. Available at: http://www.scielosp.org/scielo.php?script=sci abstract&pid=S14143 2832011000100012&lng=en&nrm=iso&tlng=es Accessed on 12/05/2016.

BRAZIL. Ministry of Health. **Comprehensive care for women's health**: bases for programmatic action. Brasilia: Ministry of Health, 1984.

BRAZIL. Ministry of Health. **Indigenous pregnant women receive special care at maternity hospital in Roraima**. 2016. Available at: http://portalsaude.saude.gov.br/ Accessed on 23/05/2016.

BRAZIL. Ministry of Health. National Health Foundation - FUNASA. **National Health Care Policy for Indigenous Peoples**. Approved by Ministry of Health Ordinance No. 254, of January 31, 2002 (Dou No. 26 - section 1, p. 46 to 49, of February 6, 2002).

BRASIL. **Política Nacional de Atençâo Integral à Saùde da Mulher**: Principios e Diretrizes. Brasilia: Ministry of Health; 2004.

COELHO, Marta Roberta S. Atençâo bàsica à saù da mulher: subsidios para a elaboração do manual do gestor municipal. Dissertation (Masters in Collective Health) - Institute of Collective Health, Federal University of Bahia, Salvador, 2003.

COSTA, Ana Maria. **Development and implementation of PAISM in Brazil**. Brasilia: NESP; CEAM; UnB, 1999. Available at: http://books.scielo.org/id/t4s9t/18 Accessed on 12/04/2016.

HAHNER, June Edith. **Emancipation of the Female Sex**: the struggle for women's rights in Brazil. 1850-1940. Florianópolis/Santa Cruz do Sul, Ed. Mulheres/EDUNISC, 2003.

MENEZES, Mariane de Oliveira. **Gestating and giving birth in the land of *Juruà***: the experience of *Guarani-mbyà* women in the city of São Paulo. Master's dissertation - University of São Paulo: School of Public Health. 2012. Available at: www.teses.usp.br/teses/disponiveis/6/6136/tde-10092012 Accessed on 25/05/2016.

MOLITERNO, Aline Cardoso Machado. Et.al. The process of pregnancy and childbirth among Kaingang women. **Texto e Contexto Enfermagem**, v.22, n° 2, Florianópolis, 2013. Available at: http://www.scielo.br/scielo.php?script=sci_arttext&pid=S0104-07072013000200004&lng=en&nrm=iso&tlng=pt Access in 22/05/2016.

LAKATOS, Eva Maria; MARCONI, Marina de Andrade. **Fundamentals of scientific methodology**: research techniques. 7 ed. São Paulo: Atlas, 2010.

13. THE DENTIST'S INTERACTION WITH INDIGENOUS COMMUNITIES AND THE CONSEQUENCES FOR ORAL HEALTH

Veronica Teresa Cardoso Zàrete, Clóvis LucianoGiacomet

INTRODUCTION

When we think about the applicability of efficient health models in an indigenous socio-cultural context, we realize that the solution must go far beyond the urgent introduction of qualified health professionals in their specialties in the villages. More precisely, when it comes to an efficient model of indigenous oral health, the problem is even worse: in addition to the fact that there is little demand for candidates for this type of demand due to the difficulties inherent in this field of activity, there is a primary need for these professionals to have a minimum idea of what they will face when they are immersed in a cross-cultural environment that will usually leave them without even the basic communication of the professional-patient relationship. It is at this point, then, that the barriers are no longer just geographical and administrative, but expand infinitely into the universe of culture. An indigenous patient brings with them their interpretation of the world around them, of life and death, of the spiritual causes of illness, of healing and, of course, a concept of their own cultural "health system".

When the health professional carries out his work treating the indigenous patient as if he were a patient from an urban context, there will be a shock, because the professional-patient relationship is different and, due to the diversity of the cultures involved, it is likely that the following will occur: (1) Disbelief on the part of the indigenous person regarding the treatment offered; (2) Non-acceptance of a continuous treatment considered "time-consuming" in the eyes of the indigenous patient because it requires several visits to the dentist; and/or (3) Failure to develop new preventive health habits.

The focus here, although not exclusively, is on the health professionals and the management team, and the proposal is to rethink their work in the village without a pre-understanding of the practical anthropological concept of culture, which would help them to better understand this intercultural dialogue, giving them more "tools" to do their job properly, resulting in a more humane, less ethnocentric and imposing service, one that is more respectful, more effective in raising awareness of the value of adequate and effective hygiene practices, and which also seeks to understand and take advantage of the local natural resources that are previously known and traditionally used by the indigenous community.

THE CLASH OF THE TWO KNOWLEDGES

In 2002, the Ministry of Education, in partnership with the General Organization of Bilingual Ticuna Teachers (OGPTB), published an oral health textbook written by the indigenous people themselves, duly advised by a team of specialists in the fields of health, specifically dentistry and education. In addition to the themes of food and chewing based on their myths and stories, the Oral Health Book presents the use of the plant called Wotch to clean teeth by the ancestors of the Ticuna people, and the use of a "dental floss" made from the leaves of the Tucumâ palm. Now, this initiative refers to the indigenous autonomy of the Ticuna, at the forefront in terms of solving their own problems, in this case toothache and its complications, and this at any time, even in pre-Columbian and pre-Cabraline America.

However, in asserting such autonomy, the first barrier to overcome is Western, modern science itself, which according to Santos (2009) is an abyssal knowledge when it ends up annulling, illegitimizing and denying any other knowledge that does not precede it. This Western epistemology is exclusionary, invisibilizing and asymmetrical in Santos'

(2009) terms with regard to traditional knowledge, and according to Narby (1997), "The Western world is unwilling to enter into a real dialogue with these peoples, since its biological science cannot receive their knowledge because of the epistemological block", which, being materialist from its historical origins, "mortifies" nature, which for indigenous people is alive and active in their cosmology.

So, taking Santos' (2009) and Narby's (1997) criticisms of modern epistemological thinking as a starting point, in which it is wrong to deny the possibility of the veracity of traditional peoples' knowledge, demeaning it and making it invisible in the face of so-called scientific knowledge, we will propose a reflection on the anteriority of this traditional knowledge to what we now call science, including dealing with toothache with the resources and techniques available to these peoples who preexisted our modern dentistry, not to belittle it, of course, but to also praise local knowledge by proposing a dialogical and symmetrical stance in the dentist-indigenous relationship in the construction of a dentistry that is more suited to the reality experienced in the villages.

THE IMPORTANCE OF TEETH FOR INDIGENOUS PEOPLE

Sousa (2010) also asserts that humans have cared for their teeth since ancient times. He attributes the invention of the modern version of the toothbrush to William Addis, a British prisoner in the 18th century, but also reports a Chinese prototype made of bamboo in 1490, and a plant branch found in a five thousand year old Egyptian tomb with one of the ends shredded in the likeness of Mohammed (570-633), the use of aromatic wood sticks to clean and whiten teeth, and various other records of the use of mint, ash, sand and even urine as means used by various native peoples in ancient times to care for teeth and breath.

Of course, teeth aren't just a source of distress and pain in the indigenous world. In their cosmovision, there are explanations for the origin of teeth, the cause of their rapid appearance or delay in babies, the cause of loss, care to be taken, etc.

According to Moimaz et al (2001), indigenous people naturally perceive the importance of oral health and teeth in chewing, appearance and oral hygiene, and associate it with the good performance of daily activities in the village. These authors, following their research in the village of Icatau, made up of indigenous people from the Kaingàng and Terena ethnic groups, in the municipality of Braùna-SP, conclude: Given the results, it can be concluded that the indigenous person's perception of health is directly related to their ability to carry out tasks in the community, just as the importance attributed to appearance and chewing ability is related to their general state of health.

Like the research by Moimaz et al (2001), the Matses language also uses their main verb for "to eat", pequin, which also means "to bite". Thus, humans and animals "bite" things or "food", pete - "that which is eaten", solid food, chewable food (MNTB, 2011 b).

This association between biting, chewing and eating exposes the awareness of the importance of the tooth in chewing their food, and since it is unnecessary to dwell on this point, we will now emphasize the relevance of its instrumental, aesthetic and warlike use in the indigenous context.

It should be noted that indigenous people have their own systems for interpreting, preventing and treating diseases. In this way, MENTA (2002) observed that the health-disease process of indigenous peoples manifests itself empirically and clearly more in the collective than in the individual sphere, and that illnesses can have different etiologies such as flight from the soul, shamanic sorcery, natural and supernatural explanations, among others. MUNAGA (2007) cited envy, revenge and punishment for breaking rules or discontent with the ancestors, gods and spirits of the family in the absence of cults as causes.

INTERETHNIC FRICTION

Indigenous patient Cardoso de Oliveira (1972), based on his fieldwork among the Tücuna in Alto Solimoes-AM in the 1960s, was the first to use the term "interethnic friction" to express the sociocultural phenomena following a tribal group's contact with national society, usually a conflictual relationship. Thirty years later, Cardoso de Oliveira (1994) comments that he didn't intend to create a concept, a "theory" about it, but that it was taken up and quoted by his own readers from that moment on.

In any case, what he really wanted was to show what happens in this contact relationship, but only in terms of "notions" of interethnic "friction". Oliveira Filho (1999) and Viveiros de Castro (1999) question Cardoso de Oliveira's (1972) perspective, especially with regard to acculturation, i.e. the idea that the Indian is doomed to lose his traditional culture as a result of asymmetrical contact with national society.

For this study specifically, it won't be necessary to dwell on the dialogue between these authors, although it is highly relevant to what is meant by inter-ethnic relations, but just to point out that although the dentist is not the first non-indigene to arrive in the village, he is still an agent in the context of inter-ethnic contact, with equipment, instruments, masks, gloves and medicines, even in some cases, These items are configured as "alien elements" and can have a cultural impact due to possible interpretations, such as, for example, among the Matses, the possibility of an association with the apparitions of spirits they call Chishcan - the dolphin - who in human form always appear bearded and wearing white robes (MNTB, 2011a). "Interethnic friction" would then be, according to Cardoso de Oliveira (1972), what happens in an interethnic contact between the health professional as an agent of national society and the indigenous person, when each sees the other's differences and from there plans their behavior based on the interpretations generated in the contact.

This is an asymmetrical and conflicting relationship in terms of objectives and ideas, in which the indigenous person ends up losing out to the detriment of their culture and traditional knowledge. Understanding that your patient's world is different from yours is essential to the success of the dental surgeon's work. There will certainly be a one-off success in terms of the clinical procedure, but are there any "tools" in their academic baggage for a relevant and lasting intervention?

ETNOCENTRISM

Ethnocentrism is a universal phenomenon. It is a common belief that society itself is the center of humanity, or even its only expression. The fundamental point of reference is not humanity, but the group. Hence the reaction, or at least the strangeness, towards foreigners. The arrival of a stranger in certain communities can be seen as a breach of the social or supernatural order.

When the interethnic encounter that takes place in the dentist-indigenous patient relationship in the village is dissociated from this compression of sociocultural reality, dental work will be doomed to the work of removing dental elements, because it is still a stranger intervening in the village routine, teaching new hygiene habits and techniques that could directly interfere with the economy, social food taboos, local hygiene modes and concept.

Based on his field experience, Manzano (2011) explains how the work of providing health care in indigenous areas is already fraught with difficulties, and that these are even more intense when it comes to the work of a CD in a village. This is because it's obviously not a question of a patient coming to a comfortable office in the city already fully equipped to serve them, but it's the office itself - fully adapted to adverse conditions - going to meet the patient.

In addition to all the difficulties involved in transporting equipment and instruments, there is also the weight of the lack of understanding of the cultural context involved. The relationship between health professionals and patients, regardless of the area in which they work, goes far beyond the application of the technical knowledge acquired during their professional training.

ETHNOCENTRISM IN THE INDIGENOUS DENTIST-PATIENT RELATIONSHIP

Ethnocentrism is another important concept in anthropology. It is literally having your ethnicity at the center. Lévi-Strauss (1993) demarginalizes the term, which until then had only been viewed negatively, by referring to it as "a natural phenomenon resulting from direct or indirect relations between societies", in other words: in some way everyone acts like this. For him, ethnocentrism "consists of purely and simply repudiating cultural forms: moral, religious, social, aesthetic, which are the most distant from those with which we identify ourselves".

Laraia (2004), in agreement, explains ethnocentrism: The fact that man sees the world through his culture results in a tendency to consider his way of life as the most correct and the most natural. This tendency, called ethnocentrism, is responsible in its extreme cases for the occurrence of numerous social conflicts. According to Laraia (2004), this attitude of measuring the other, the different, not on the basis of humanity in all its diversity, but on the basis of one's own group, ethnicity, local values, ideals and morals, is "a universal phenomenon". It would therefore be naïve not to understand that this phenomenon also occurs in the dentist-indigenous patient relationship on the occasion of interethnic contact. Fourniol Filho (1981) speaks in terms of an organic reaction when he states that: The nervous system, the internal secretion glands and environmental factors regulate the balance of our organism.

Whatever the nature of the stimulus, our body will respond to the aggression. The reaction triggered depends on the intensity of the aggressor and the balance of the organism will be modified. This reaction is called BEHAVIOR or CONDUCT. And the Indian's conduct is evident in this situation. As observed by Dias (2011) in the Alto Javari, in a Matses community, in the decade 1997-2007, health professionals undertook great juggling acts in an effort to communicate with their Matses patients, albeit precariously through gestures, due to their little or no understanding of the national language - and also of the native language by the health professional - sometimes trying to explain quantities of medicine to take (drops or tablets), or the time and for how many days to take the medicine; or explaining hygiene and grooming notions for children; or giving notions of brushing, oral hygiene, or the typical application of fluoride.

What might have seemed to the professionals to be a way of making up for the "limited or diminished capacity to understand" of the indigenous patients, who were sometimes treated like children, was comical for the Matses. Usually, disagreements, laughter and debauched jokes from the group in the Matses language - never translated into Portuguese by the native in charge - took place between them during the health professional's lecture. Interethnic contact will always bring out a certain ethnocentric reaction, which is peculiar to human nature. In agreement with this, Rivière (2007, p. 13) says that "it is natural to every human being" and "everyone has a tendency to reject, criticize or devalue those who are not like them", and exemplifies and conceptualizes this: When America was discovered, the Spanish initially rejected the character of humanity of the Indians, sometimes to justify slavery; on the other hand, the Indians killed Spaniards to prove that they really were mortal. Ethnocentrism, which the ethnologist tries to get rid of, is the attitude that consists of judging the moral, religious and social forms of other communities according to our own standards and, therefore, considering their differences as an anomaly. Rivière (2007) also differentiates between ethnocentrism and racism. Reaction to the exotic is ethnocentrism when it expresses devaluation of the other, and it is racism when it produces "rejection and hostility".

Laraia (2004) mitigates the negativity of reactionary human ethnocentrism by treating Apathy as its antonym - which reflects a negative attitude towards one's own ethnicity, resulting in a greater evil, since "instead of overestimating the values of their own society, in a given crisis situation the members of a culture abandon their belief in these values and consequently lose the motivation that keeps them united and alive". Since the indigenous patient and the health professional come from different worlds, in some cases, as in the Javari Valley, also using different languages, it is natural for each to measure the other from their own cultural paradigms. At this point, we can think of the Matses/Mayoruna nomenclature as an example, which discriminates/classifies men into three groups: Matses (when they refer to themselves, their ethnicity. It means "people"; a Mayoruna, people in the sense of human - not animal); Matses utsi ("other people". They use this expression for other indigenous groups in the region) and Chotac, the Naua, the white man, the foreigner (MATOS, 2009). Yuca bishuccaid - "peeled yuca" (MNTB, 2011a) is their typical joke, comparing truly white people to yuca when peeled, because it is all white inside.

The comments of Tuiâvii, chief of the Trivéia tribe in Polynesia, published by Scheurmann (2003) under the title O Papalagui, also show the above, when after a period in Europe, Tuiâvii, returning to his people, tells what he saw about the way of life, the clothing, the housing, the ambitions, the oppression of the lack of time, the hollow religiosity etc. of the Europeans.

Scheurmann's (2003) intention in publishing these comments was to give Europeans a self-portrait, a view of themselves through the eyes of a man considered "primitive", exhorting his people on a distant island never to become like the white Papalagui. Darcy Ribeiro is also surprising when, in his book O povo brasileiro (The Brazilian People), he conjures up the Indian's perspective on meeting the "bearded", "smelly" Portuguese, locked up in their boats for months at sea... and who still thought the Indian was dirty and lazy! In the book Os indios e a civilização (RIBEIRO, 1996), the perspective of the Indian (Kaingang - from São Paulo; Xokleng; Parintintin) in contact with the officials of the now defunct SPI (Indian Protection Service) is presented. Ribeiro explains that it was the Indian who always took the initiative to contact the white man, to "tame" him, to be more precise. For those people, "ferocious animals" and "perverse by instinct" - expressions directed at the Kayapó by the sertanejos, in reality, it was the Whites who were the "savages" who needed to be tamed, and the massacre of the Cinta-Larga (Ji-Paranâ) by the "civilized" narrated on pages 209 and 210 (mass shooting, cowardice and rape) vehemently confirms the Indians' thesis. Therefore, properly equipped with a relativistic predisposition when dealing with indigenous patients, health professionals will be able to understand the impact of their presence, as well as their service and all the technology used in the context, and deal with reactions in an understanding way, also investing their time in a symmetrical dialogue with the indigenous person to solve the community's oral health problems, in which both will certainly be interested and committed.

THE IMPORTANCE OF LISTENING: A CONTRIBUTION FROM ETHNO-PSYCHOLOGY

In view of the above, it is important to emphasize that ethnopsychology can contribute to the aforementioned meetings for the preparation of future dental surgeons and go further by shedding light on a new therapeutic approach to be developed by these professionals, such as the one below.

Two psychoanalytic concepts borrowed from psychoanalysis can play an important role in this discussion: the other, according to BAIRRÂO (1999), refers to the symbolic heritage, which is generic to humanity and peculiar to each subject.

It is thanks to this that culture and the subject can be dealt with without ruptures, because its smallest elements, the signifiers, can at the same time have more universal implications and more subtly singular ones, depending on the particular way in which they affect each person. In this sense, in a multidisciplinary team, the ethnopsychologist's presence must be oriented towards developing intervention models that are not restricted to the individual psyche, but are also not reduced to sociological generalities (BAIRRAO, 2005). According to the same author, in psychoanalysis, the professional must always be aware of the desire of the other and their implication in this relationship of otherness.

The dental surgeon must sharpen his listening skills in order to "(...) rescue the enunciative dimension of things in cultural reality" (BAIRRAO, 2005).) rescuing its enunciative dimension in the things of cultural reality" (BAIRRAO, 2005), rescuing collective voices, restoring hidden riches to the community in which they are inserted (in professional dental activity), not overpowering the voice of the other, but, on the contrary, amplifying it, giving it reach and, finally, cultivating respect and care in listening to all the ways in which they (the other) tell themselves (and especially the less obvious ones) (BAIRRAO, 2005).

CONCLUSION

What is proposed here, in the light of the reference expressed in the text, are elements that are not exceptionally new, not least because of the existence of publications by traditional and indigenous populations on their local knowledge, including in the area of oral health, such as The Oral Health Book of the Ticuna of the Alto Solimoes by the OGPTB, which also maintains a website showing more of the culture and events of this ethnic group. In fact, not only for this study, but also for the production of other academic works, there was a significant contribution of ethnographic and socio-cultural data found on the websites and blogs of native organizations and associations that represent their people and are increasingly opening up to the virtual world.

In this sense, the main objective of this work is to emphasize the "broadening" of this awareness, which has already been awakened to a certain extent, with a view to an urgent dialogical relationship of knowledge and an anthropological reflection on what is meant by talking to indigenous people about oral hygiene, so that we can seek - and achieve - , a more efficient hygiene and prevention practice in the villages, which will only happen when the indigenous person stops being a mere "object" of the government's health programs and becomes a "subject" in them, similar to what Hountondji (2009) pointed out in the context of Africa, highlighting the speech of African authors about their own people. It is therefore only fitting that indigenous people should be heard about their own social problems ("social" because oral health is part and symptom of this whole), from their perspective, and their ideas on how to solve them. As for the academic training of dental surgeons, also presented in this text, it is not disputed that all the institutions that train dental surgeons in Brazil meet the legal requirements of the MEC.

The vast majority of these professionals are graduates of the highest technical ability and scientific rigor, prepared to work in extremely competitive contexts and also trained in the latest technologies discovered every day in a globalized world. And everyone, in some way, is looking for something to set them apart from the crowd of professionals. The hook that was sought, however, based on observations such as those by Zanetti (2007) and Reyes (2011) and especially in the text of the DCN itself, was the direction of technical and scientific rigor based on ethics and legality, with an understanding of the social, cultural and economic reality of the environment in which this professional will be inserted. In this sense, there is a need for greater investment in subjects that prepare this professional to work in different cultures, such as among indigenous peoples and traditional populations in Brazil. A few institutions, in a timid way, have subjects in their curricula that focus on the social sciences, but only as general basic training subjects.

It is therefore necessary to make interdisciplinary dialogue possible and real, as suggested by Zanetti (2007) in the text, by giving more space and relevance in the Dentistry curriculum, especially Anthropology, which, as we have tried to show in this work, has a highly relevant role to play in this issue, as it deals directly with these peoples and with themes such as culture, ethnocentrism, assimilation, interethnic contact and others discussed here. Thus, miraculous and expensive emergency alternatives such as sporadic S.O.S. campaigns and a flood of oral hygiene material in the villages, which neither produced nor will produce the desired effects for the health bodies and agencies, would be replaced by the gradual and anthropologically oriented application of dentistry enriched by traditional indigenous knowledge to the problems of tooth decay, periodontal disease and tooth loss in the villages. The result of listening to indigenous people about oral health in partnership with a dental surgeon, properly prepared for this specific target group, could only be the "expansion" of endogenous and practical guide material such as The Ticuna Oral Health Book, cited in this work. It's possible that a more technical reader will be wary of this proposal, because scientific knowledge, as Santos (2009) and Quijano (2009) have pointed out, presents itself as more precise and complete, reducing or making local knowledge invisible, making a symmetrical relationship of knowledge and people impossible, usually praising one and despising the others, making the indigenous person out to be illiterate, ignorant, superstitious, and other undesirable adjectives.

And so it may seem that we have acted with a certain irresponsibility in praising this local knowledge, but a more detailed reading of the reference used in this work would certainly lead to an anthropologically oriented, no less technical, view of the other. Anthropologists don't "invent" theories and then go into the field to check them out, like laboratory guinea pigs. They go into the field first and then narrate what they learned there, two very distinct phases of anthropological work, as Geertz (1989) wrote in his article on Being there and writing here. That's right: it's what they "learned" there, living in sociocultural contexts different from their own. This justifies the zeal for local knowledge and the defense of their space in the relationship with the non-indigenous world. This is the case of Narby (1997), also cited in this work, who raises many questions about the medicinal knowledge of the Shipibo and Ashaninka (both from the Peruvian Amazon), which he treats as too complex to have been learned through adventurous experimentation, like a lottery, by combining medicinal plants in a short period of time in which the patient can wait.

Santos' (2009) Ecology of Knowledges thus emerges as a current, scientifically correct and completely plausible proposal for application in the indigenous and traditional context. Finally, what has been exposed in this work is also the result of situations experienced by the authors in the field of Anthropology and Dentistry, and which, although separated in this period by thousands of kilometers, saw the same issues arise that they now materialize. Thus, the authors' main contribution is to verify the need for change on the part of the professional, so that the local culture can be respected and the work carried out can be relevant and lasting. And also the expectation of seeing these two types of knowledge working together to solve the oral health problems of indigenous peoples. And if it is possible to dare even more, I would also suggest extending this anthropological perspective to other areas of knowledge which, like dentistry, deal directly with indigenous and traditional peoples, but still lack this awareness of adapting to the reality of these peoples, erring with them with the same colonialism and Eurocentric scientificism that has historically led so many peoples to ethnocide.

REFERENCES

ABREU, Cathia. Toothache in the village? Rio de Janeiro: Instituto Ciência Hoje, 2005. Available at: Acesso em: 09 mar. 2011.

ACUNA, Cristobal de. New Discovery of the Great Amazon River. In: CARVAJAL, Gaspar de; ROJAS, Alonso de;. Discoveries of the Amazon River - Translated and annotated by C. de Melo Leitao. Sao Paulo: Companhia Editora Nacional, 1941. p.125-295.

ARANTES, Rui. Oral health of the indigenous peoples of Brazil and the case of the Xavante of Mato Grosso. 2005. 135 f. Thesis (Doctorate) - Ministry of Health - Oswaldo Cruz Foundation - Sérgio Arouca National School of Public Health. Rio de Janeiro, 2005.

BAIRRAO, J. F. M. H. Santa Barbara and the diva. Boleitim Formaçao em Psicanalise,v. 8, n. 1, p. 25- 38, 1999

BAIRRAO, J. F. M. A escuta participante como participante como procedimento de pesquisa do sagrado enunciante. Estudos de Psicanalise, Natal, v. 3, n. 10, p. 441- 446, 2005.

MENTA SA. The health-disease process among Brazilian populations: a conceptual and instrumental question. Tellus, 2(2): 65-72, 2002.

MOIMAZ, Suzely Adas Saliba; SALIBA, Nemre Adas; GARBIN MUMANGA K. Health and diversity. Health & Society 16(2): 1315, 2007.

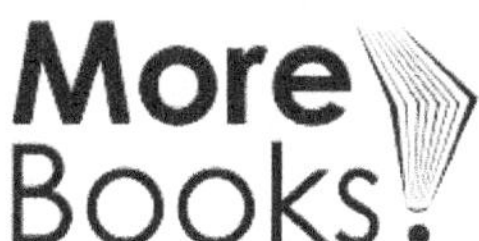

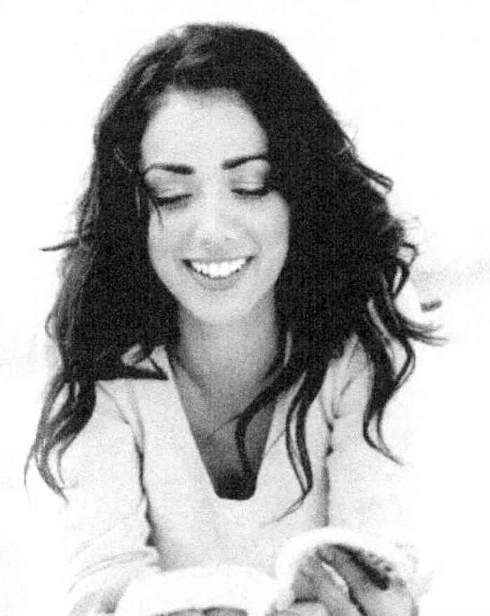

I want morebooks!

Buy your books fast and straightforward online - at one of world's fastest growing online book stores! Environmentally sound due to Print-on-Demand technologies.

Buy your books online at
www.morebooks.shop

Kaufen Sie Ihre Bücher schnell und unkompliziert online – auf einer der am schnellsten wachsenden Buchhandelsplattformen weltweit! Dank Print-On-Demand umwelt- und ressourcenschonend produziert.

Bücher schneller online kaufen
www.morebooks.shop

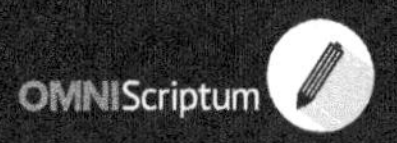

Made in the USA
Monee, IL
07 July 2026

56549914R00115